Concise
DENTAL ANATOMY
and
MORPHOLOGY

——— *Fourth Edition* ———

JAMES L. FULLER, D.D.S., M.S.

Professor Emeritus, Department of Operative Dentistry
University of Iowa College of Dentistry, Iowa City

GERALD E. DENEHY, D.D.S., M.S.

Professor, Department of Operative Dentistry
University of Iowa College of Dentistry, Iowa City

THOMAS M. SCHULEIN, D.D.S., M.S.

Associate Professor, Department of Operative Dentistry
University of Iowa College of Dentistry, Iowa City

*Illustrated by William Girsch, D.D.S.
and James Herd, B.F.A.*

Library of Congress Cataloging-in-Publication Data

Fuller, James L.

Concise dental anatomy and morphology / James L. Fuller, Gerald E. Denehy, Thomas M. Schulein ; illustrated by William Girsch and James Herd.-- 4th ed.

p. ; cm.

Includes bibliographical references and index.

ISBN 0-87414-125-7 (pbk. : alk. paper)

1. Teeth--Anatomy. I. Denehy, Gerald E. II. Schulein, Thomas M., 1945- III. Title.

[DNLM: 1. Tooth--anatomy & histology--Outlines. 2. Dentition--Outlines. WU 18.2 F966c 2001]

QM311 .F84 2001

611'.314--dc21

2001041473

PREFACE

This textbook, like most others, was prepared to conform to specific purposes. Foremost among these aims was: 1) An attempt to reduce the content, in comparison to traditional textbooks in the field, and 2) The desire to produce self-paced and self-study materials which would be compatible with recent trends in dental education toward individualized and flexible curricula.

The precursor to this formally published text was a manual intended solely for dental students. Since all dental school curricula feature in-depth courses in occlusion, histology, anatomy, physiology, etc., this manual only highlighted some of the major premises of these courses, with no attempt to duplicate their detail. It became apparent that this condensed manual was not only appropriate for dental students, but was also suitable for use in dental hygiene and dental assistant educational programs. In all of these curricula, the course in dental anatomy is normally situated first, so that it is a prerequisite for all future dental science course work. Therefore, the present text presents a basic core of material, which, if mastered by the student, will provide essential and sufficient knowledge of dental anatomy for further dental educational experiences.

The original manual was prepared in an outline form, and because of the preference of the authors, as well as encouragement from reviewers, that format has remained. Former students have also generally favored the outline format over the traditional free-flowing style.

The content is divided into eleven units, each of which can be considered as a unit of material for self-study purposes. The specific objectives which accompany each unit should serve as a study guide for the student, as well as a guide for the preparation of examinations by the instructor. Each unit is important, but many of the practical concepts presented in Unit #2 are essential to the successful practice of dentistry and dental hygiene.

It is important that the student of dental anatomy make thorough use of the text illustrations, as well as any models, dentoforms, or extracted teeth which are accessible, or provided by the course instructor. The student seems to retain the material much longer if each item under consideration is referred to a diagram or model. In this manner, the student builds a mental image of a tooth, a surface, or some other structure, which is more permanent than a mere memorization of definitions and descriptions.

Inasmuch as your course may not contain any formal lectures, experience has revealed that students who don't have the opportunity to hear unfamiliar terms pronounced correctly tend to mispronounce them. Therefore, a pronunciation guide is included at the back of the text.

For most of you, this course is the beginning of your formal studies in the dental health care field. It is the sincere hope of the authors that your participation in this profession, whatever your niche may be, will in some way make the world a better place in which to live.

JAMES L. FULLER
GERALD E. DENEHY
THOMAS M. SCHULEIN

CONTENTS

UNIT #1

I. **Reading Assignment:**

Preface

Unit #1 (Introduction and Nomenclature)

II. **Specific Objectives:**

At the completion of this unit, the student will be able to:

A.   Identify either deciduous or permanent teeth by their proper name, when given a diagram or description of their function, arch position, or alternative name. Furthermore, the student should be able to identify the type and number of deciduous or permanent teeth per quadrant, arch, and in total. Finally, the student should be able to identify the type and number of teeth which are anterior or posterior.

B.   Provide the proper definition, or select the correct definition or description from a list, for any structure presented in the sections covering general anatomy and anatomical structures. Furthermore, the student should be able to make applications of these terms to diagrams or situations.

C.   Demonstrate a knowledge of dental formulae by supplying, or selecting from a list, the correct information regarding a given dental formula.

D.   Indicate the normal eruption sequence, or order, for deciduous and permanent teeth, by listing, or selecting from a list, the proper sequences.

E.   Define, or correctly identify from a list, the three periods of man's dentition, as well as identify the approximate time intervals of their existence, and normal initiation and termination events.

F.   Define the term "succedaneous", and be able to select from a list the tooth or teeth which are succedaneous.

G.   Identify, or select from a list, the proper name for tooth surfaces, or thirds of tooth surfaces, when given a diagram or description.

H.   Select the correct answer from a list, or supply the correct name, for line or point angles, when given a diagram or description.

I.   Demonstrate knowledge of the various dental numbering systems presented, by supplying, or selecting from a list, the correct name or description for a given symbol, or the correct symbol for a given name or description.

J.   Provide, or select from a list, the correct definition, or application thereof, for any of the dentition classifications studied.

K.   Provide, or select from a list, the correct definition of any underlined term not included in any previous objective. Furthermore, the student will be able to make applications of these terms to descriptions, diagrams, or situations.

UNIT #1
INTRODUCTION AND NOMENCLATURE

I. **Introduction:**

A.   The teeth are arranged in upper and lower <u>arches</u>. Those teeth in the upper arch are termed <u>maxillary</u>, because they are set in the upper jaw, which is the <u>maxilla</u> (Plural - maxillae). The teeth in the lower arch are termed <u>mandibular</u>, because they are located in the lower jaw, which is the <u>mandible</u>. The mandible is the movable member of the two jaws, while the maxilla is stationary.

B.   The imaginary vertical line which divides each arch, as well as the body, into two approximately equal halves, is the <u>midline</u>. Strictly speaking, this vertical division is not a one-dimensional line at all, but rather a two-dimensional plane, termed the <u>mid-sagittal plane</u>. However, since most dental authors persist in using the less appropriate term "midline", for consistency this text will also use it. The two approximately equal portions of each arch divided by the midline are termed <u>quadrants</u>, since there are four in the entire mouth. They are termed:

maxillary (upper) right.

maxillary (upper) left.

mandibular (lower) right.

mandibular (lower) left.

C.   It is important to point out that as one looks directly at the oral cavity (or the body) from the front, the anatomical directions of right and left are reversed. Hence, the right side of the mouth is actually to the left of the viewer, while the left side of the mouth is to the right of the viewer.

D.   The manner in which the mandibular teeth contact the maxillary teeth is called <u>occlusion</u>. The term for the process of biting or chewing of food is <u>mastication</u>.

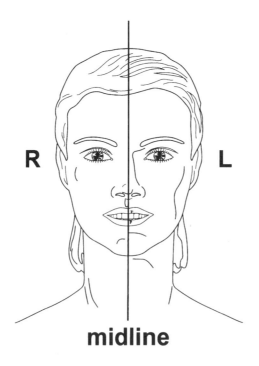

midline

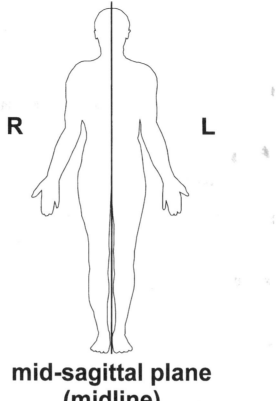

mid-sagittal plane (midline)

II. Classification of Dentitions:

A. The human dentition is termed heterodont, which means it is comprised of different types, or classes, of teeth to perform different functions in the mastication process. In comparison, a homodont dentition is one in which all of the teeth are the same in form and type. This sort of dentition is found in some of the lower vertebrates.

B. Furthermore, man has two separate sets of teeth, or dentitions. This is termed diphyodont, as opposed to monophyodont, when there is only one set of teeth, and polyphyodont, when more than two, or continuous, sets of teeth are developed throughout life.

C. In man, the two dentitions are termed deciduous and permanent, while the transitional phase when both deciduous and permanent teeth are present is called the mixed dentition period.

  1. Deciduous dentition - The teeth of the first, or primary dentition. They are so named because they are shed like the leaves of deciduous trees in autumn. They erupt into the mouth from about six months to two years of age. Normally there are 20 total deciduous teeth. Other non-scientific names for the deciduous teeth include "milk" teeth, "baby" teeth, and "temporary" teeth.

  2. Permanent dentition - The teeth of the second, or adult dentition. Normally, there are 32 permanent teeth and they erupt from 6-21 years of age.

III. Classification of the Teeth:

A.   Permanent Dentition:

As was pointed out, man is a heterodont, which means that more than one type of tooth is found in the human dentitions. Each complete quadrant of the permanent dentition contains eight teeth of differing type and function, as follows:

1.   Incisors (2) - The incisors are the two teeth of each quadrant which are closest to the midline. They are named central and lateral incisors. Their functions in mastication are biting, cutting, incising and shearing. There are four permanent incisors per arch, and a total of eight in the mouth.

2.   Canine (1) - The canine is the third tooth from the midline in each quadrant. Its function in mastication is cutting, tearing, piercing, and holding. It also is called a cuspid. There are two permanent canines per arch, and a total of four in the mouth.

3.   Premolars (2) - The premolars are the fourth and fifth teeth from the midline. They are termed first and second premolars. Their masticatory role is tearing, holding, and grinding. They are also called bicuspids. As with the incisors, there are four per arch, and eight total premolars.

4.   Molars (3) - The molars are the sixth, seventh, and eighth teeth from the midline. They are termed first, second, and third molars. They are also called six year molar, twelve year molar, and wisdom tooth, in that order. Their masticatory function is grinding. There are six permanent molars per arch, and twelve total permanent molars.

It can thus be seen that there are 16 permanent teeth in a complete arch, and a total of 32 teeth in the permanent dentition.

B.   Deciduous Dentition:

Each quadrant of man's deciduous dentition contains the following types of teeth, all of which have a function similar to their permanent complements:

1.   Incisors (2), which are named central and lateral incisors.

2.   Canine (1), or cuspid.

3.   Molars (2), which are named first and second molars.

Therefore, there are five deciduous teeth per quadrant, ten per arch, and a total of twenty in the primary dentition. When compared to the permanent teeth, the primary dentition contains an identical number of incisors and canines, but has no premolars and one less molar per quadrant.

IV. Dentition Periods and Succedaneous Teeth:

A.   It has been pointed out that man has two dentitions, but three periods of dentition, since the deciduous and permanent dentitions overlap in time. These periods are summarized in the following manner:

1.   Primary dentition period - That period during which only deciduous teeth are present, and occurs from approximately six months to six years of age. The primary dentition period ends at about age six, with the eruption of the first permanent tooth, normally the mandibular first molar.

2.   Mixed dentition period - That period during which both deciduous and permanent teeth are present, and lasts from approximately six years to twelve years of age. The mixed dentition period ends and the permanent dentition period begins around age twelve, with the exfoliation of the last deciduous tooth, normally the maxillary second molar.

DENTITION STAGES

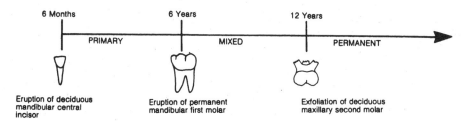

3. <u>Permanent dentition period</u> - That period when only permanent teeth are present, and which begins at approximately twelve years of age and continues through the rest of life.

B. In order for a permanent tooth to erupt into a space where a deciduous tooth is located, the deciduous tooth must first be shed, or exfoliated. The natural process by which deciduous roots are "melted away" to allow for exfoliation is termed resorption.

C. Permanent teeth that replace exfoliated deciduous teeth are called succedaneous teeth, which simply means "succeeding" deciduous teeth. Since there are twenty deciduous teeth to be replaced, there must be twenty succedaneous teeth. The permanent teeth that are also succedaneous teeth include the incisors and canines, which replace their deciduous counterparts, and the premolars, which replace the deciduous molars. Therefore, the only permanent teeth which are not succedaneous are the molars. It may be said, then, that all succedaneous teeth are permanent teeth, but all permanent teeth are not succedaneous teeth.

V. Dental Formulae:

A. Dental formula - A number and letter designation of the various types of teeth found in a dentition. The dental formula indicates the dentition of only one side of the mouth, but includes both the upper and lower quadrants, and so must be multiplied by a factor of two to provide the number of teeth in the entire dentition.

B. Thus, the dental formula for man's permanent dentition is as follows:

$$I - \frac{2}{2} : C - \frac{1}{1} : P - \frac{2}{2} : M - \frac{3}{3} \text{ (x 2 = 32 total teeth)}$$

C. The deciduous dentition of man has the following dental formula:

$$I - \frac{2}{2} : C - \frac{1}{1} : M - \frac{2}{2} \text{ (x 2 = 20 total teeth)}$$

It should be kept in mind that animals other than man may have differing dental formulae.

VI. General Eruption Pattern:

Both the deciduous and permanent dentitions have a general order, or pattern, of eruption. For the deciduous dentition, this pattern normally is as follows:

A. Deciduous Dentition: Normal Eruption Sequence

   1. Mandibular central incisor

   2. Mandibular lateral incisor

3. Maxillary central incisor
4. Maxillary lateral incisor
5. Mandibular first molar
6. Maxillary first molar
7. Mandibular canine
8. Maxillary canine
9. Mandibular second molar
10. Maxillary second molar

As a general rule, mandibular deciduous teeth normally precede their maxillary counterparts in eruption. It can also be said that the deciduous teeth normally erupt in order from the front of the mouth toward the back, even though the canines in each quadrant normally erupt after the first molars.

B. Deciduous Dentition: Normal Eruption Time

Eruption Age (Months)				
	Mandible	Order	Maxilla	Order
Central Incisor	6	1	7 $\frac{1}{2}$	1
Lateral Incisor	7	2	9	2
Canine	16	4	19	4
First Molar	12	3	14	3
Second Molar	20	5	24	5

C. Permanent Dentition: Normal Eruption Sequence
1. Mandibular first molar
2. Maxillary first molar
3. Mandibular central incisor
4. Mandibular lateral incisor
5. Maxillary central incisor
6. Maxillary lateral incisor
7. Mandibular canine
8. Mandibular first premolar
9. Maxillary first premolar
10. Mandibular second premolar
11. Maxillary second premolar
12. Maxillary canine
13. Mandibular second molar
14. Maxillary second molar
15. Mandibular third molar
16. Maxillary third molar

As can be seen, the permanent mandibular teeth normally precede their maxillary counterparts in eruption, as was also the pattern with the deciduous teeth. If the first molar's eruption sequence is ignored, the permanent mandibular teeth exhibit a perfect anterior to posterior order. However, in the maxillary arch, not only is the first molar out of order, but the canine normally follows both premolars.

D. Permanent Dentition: Normal Eruption Time

	Eruption Age (Years)			
	Mandible	Order	Maxilla	Order
Central Incisor	6-7	2	7-8	2
Lateral Incisor	7-8	3	8-9	3
Canine	9-10	4	11-12	6
First Premolar	10-11	5	10-11	4
Second Premolar	11-12	6	11-12	5
First Molar	6-7	1	6-7	1
Second Molar	11-13	7	12-13	7
Third Molar	17-21	8	17-21	8

E. It should be noted that the eruption sequences and dates presented here are based on the only studies available, which were conducted a number of years ago. More contemporary data has suggested that, in some cases, these figures may not be entirely correct. It has also been suggested that there really may not be a "normal" eruption pattern which is true for both sexes, and across all racial groups. In other words, the most common eruption sequences may occur in only a relatively small percentage of the total population. However, until the results of longitudinal studies for North American populations are available, "old" sequences and dates will be used.

VII.   Numbering Systems:

Numbering systems in dentistry serve as abbreviations. Instead of writing out the entire name of a tooth, such as permanent maxillary right central incisor, it is much simpler to assign it a number, letter, or symbol, such as #8 for the universal numbering system. Of the many systems, the three most commonly used will be described.

A. Universal Numbering System:

The numbering system which enjoys the widest use today is the universal system. It employs a different number (1-32) in a consecutive arrangement for all permanent teeth, and a number-letter (1d-20d) for each of the deciduous teeth.

1.   Permanent Teeth - The universal numbering system assigns a specific number to each permanent tooth. The upper right third molar is #1, the upper right second molar #2, and so forth around the entire maxillary arch to the upper left third molar, which is #16. Since there are no more permanent teeth in the maxillary arch, the succession drops to the lower left third molar which is #17, and continues around the entire mandibular arch where the lower right third molar is #32. For example, tooth #11 is the permanent maxillary left canine.

2.   Deciduous Teeth - The twenty teeth of the deciduous dentition are numbered in the same manner as are the permanent teeth (1-20), except that a small (d) is added as a suffix to each number to designate deciduous. The deciduous upper right second molar is thus #1d, while the upper left second molar is #10d. The lower right canine, for example, is #18d.

The most common system in use today for designating deciduous teeth uses the capital letters A through T. The maxillary right deciduous second molar is tooth A and the order progresses in the manner used with the 1-32 system for permanent teeth, so that the mandibular right deciduous second molar is tooth T.

B. Palmer Notation Method:

Another commonly used numerical and letter notation scheme for identifying an individual tooth utilizes a simple symbol, which differs for each of the four quadrants. In addition, the numbers 1 through 8 are used to identify permanent central incisor through third molar in the specified quadrant. Letters A through E, with the quadrant symbol, are used for the deciduous dentition.

DECIDUOUS DENTITION

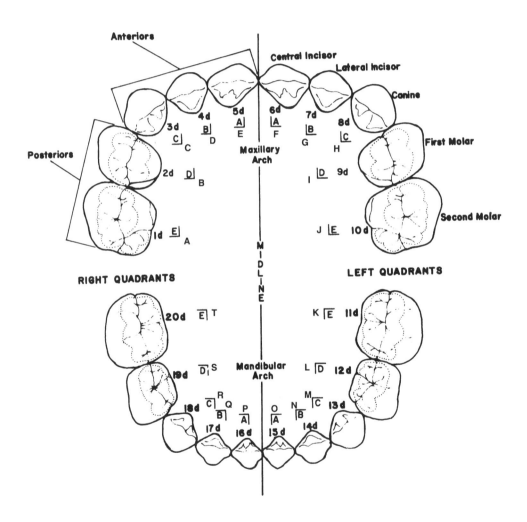

PERMANENT DENTITION

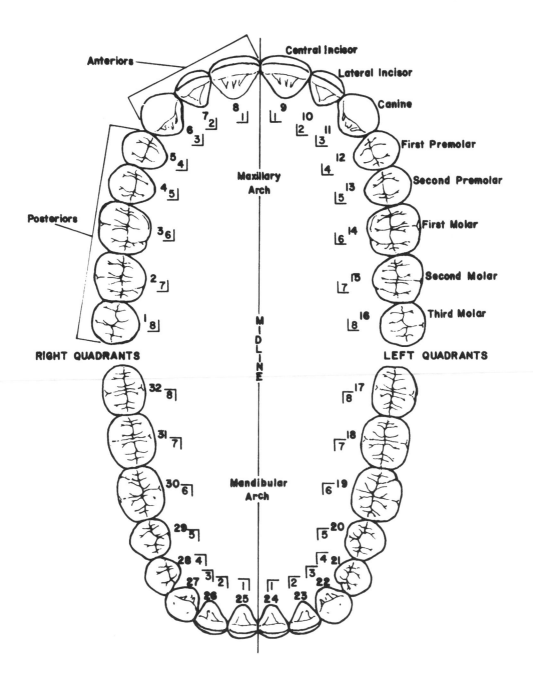

Anteriors

Central Incisor

Lateral Incisor

Canine

First Premolar

Second Premolar

First Molar

Second Molar

Third Molar

Posteriors

Maxillary Arch

MIDLINE

RIGHT QUADRANTS

LEFT QUADRANTS

Mendibular Arch

9

MAXILLARY

	E	D	C	B	A	A	B	C	D	E		
8	7	6	5	4	3	2	1	1	2	3	4	5	6	7	8

Right ———————————————————— Left

8	7	6	5	4	3	2	1	1	2	3	4	5	6	7	8
	E	D	C	B	A	A	B	C	D	E		

MANDIBULAR

Specific examples are:

6| Permanent maxillary right first molar

|3   Permanent maxillary left canine

|B   Deciduous mandibular left lateral incisor

4| Permanent mandibular right first premolar

C. FDI System:

The Federation Dentaire Internationale (FDI), the international dental organization, has introduced a new numbering system, which is an attempt at standardization throughout the world. Although presently not in worldwide use, it may be in the future. It is a simple binomial system, which includes both permanent and deciduous teeth. The first of the two numbers identifies the quadrant, and whether the tooth is permanent or deciduous, as follows:

1 - Permanent maxillary right quadrant

2 - Permanent maxillary left quadrant

3 - Permanent mandibular left quadrant

4 - Permanent mandibular right quadrant

5 - Deciduous maxillary right quadrant

6 - Deciduous maxillary left quadrant

7 - Deciduous mandibular left quadrant

8 - Deciduous mandibular right quadrant

The second number identifies the particular tooth in the quadrant, exactly like the Palmer notation method for permanent teeth (1-8). The deciduous teeth in each quadrant are numbered (1-5), the number increasing in size from the midline posteriorly.

Examples in notation utilizing the FDI system are as follows:

18 - Permanent maxillary right third molar

27 - Permanent maxillary left second molar

36 - Permanent mandibular left first molar

45 - Permanent mandibular right second premolar

54 - Deciduous maxillary right first molar

63 - Deciduous maxillary left canine

72 - Deciduous mandibular left lateral incisor

81 - Deciduous mandibular right central incisor

As review, the first designation in the above list (18) can be analyzed as follows:

1–The first number indicates that the tooth is located in the permanent maxillary right quadrant.

8–The second number indicates that the tooth is eighth from the midline, and thus is a third molar.

VIII. General Oral and Dental Anatomy:

A brief definition and description of the various anatomical features of a normal tooth, and its supporting structures, include the following:

A. Dental Structures:

1. <u>Anatomical crown</u> - That portion of the tooth which is covered by enamel.

2. <u>Clinical crown</u> - That portion of the tooth which is visible in the mouth. The clinical crown may, or may not, correspond to the anatomical crown, depending on the level of the tooth's investing soft tissue, and so may also include a portion of the anatomical root. As can be seen from this description, the clinical crown may be an ever changing entity throughout life, while the anatomical crown is a constant entity.

3. <u>Anatomical root</u> - That portion of the tooth which is covered with cementum.

4. <u>Clinical root</u> - That portion of the tooth which is not visible in the mouth. Again, the clinical root is an ever changing entity, and may, or may not, correspond to the anatomical root.

Note: In the dental literature, the modifying terms "clinical" and "anatomical" are not often used with crown or root, but the intended meaning is most often "anatomical" and so will be used in this manner hereafter.

5. <u>Enamel</u> - The hard, mineralized tissue which covers the dentin of the anatomical crown of a tooth. It is the hardest living body tissue, but is brittle, especially when not supported by sound underlying dentin.

6. <u>Dentin</u> - The hard tissue which forms the main body of the tooth. It surrounds the pulp cavity, and is covered by the enamel in the anatomical crown, and by the cementum in the anatomical root. The dentin constitutes the bulk, or majority, of the total tooth tissues, but because of its internal location, is not directly visible in a normal tooth.

7. <u>Cementum</u> - The layer of hard, bonelike tissue which covers the dentin of the anatomical root of a tooth.

8. <u>Cervical line</u> - The identifiable line around the external surface of a tooth where the enamel and cementum meet. It is also called the <u>cemento-enamel junction</u> or <u>CEJ</u>. The cervical line separates the anatomical crown and the anatomical root, and is a constant entity. Its location is in the general area of the tooth spoken of as the <u>neck</u> or <u>cervix</u>.

9. <u>Dentino-enamel junction</u> or <u>DEJ</u> - The internal line of meeting of the dentin and enamel in the anatomical crown of a tooth.

10. <u>Pulp</u> - The living soft tissue which occupies the pulp cavity of a vital tooth. It contains the tooth's nutrient supply in the form of blood vessels, as well as the nerve supply.

11. <u>Pulp Cavity</u> - The entire internal cavity of a tooth which contains the pulp. It consists of the following entities:

a. <u>Pulp canal(s)</u> - That portion of the pulp cavity which is located in the root(s) of the tooth, and may also be called the root canal(s).

11

b. Pulp chamber - The enlarged portion of the pulp cavity which is found mostly in the anatomical crown of the tooth.

c. Pulp horns - The usually pointed incisal or occlusal elongations of the pulp chamber which often correspond to the cusps, or lobes of the teeth.

B. Supporting Structures:

1. Alveolar process - The entire bony entity which surrounds and supports all the teeth in each jaw member.

2. Alveolus (Plural - alveoli) - The bony socket, or portion of the alveolar process, into which an individual tooth is set.

3. Periodontal ligament (membrane) - The fibrous attachment of the tooth cementum to the alveolar bone.

4. Gingiva (Plural - gingivae) - The "gum" or "gums", or the fibrous tissue enclosed by mucous membrane that covers the alveolar processes and surrounds the necks of the teeth.

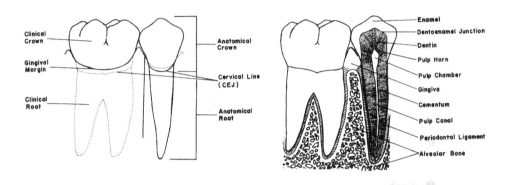

IX. Dental Nomenclature:

It is imperative that the same terms are consistently used for the various anatomical areas of the teeth, so that the dental health team can converse in a precise but simple manner. The following, then, is a portion of this common language of dentistry:

A. Anterior teeth - The teeth in either arch which are toward the front of the mouth. In both the deciduous and permanent dentitions, the anterior teeth include the incisors and canines, a total of three per quadrant and twelve in all.

B. Posterior teeth - The teeth in either arch which are toward the back of the mouth. In the deciduous dentition, this includes the two molars in each quadrant, or a total of eight teeth. In the permanent dentition, this includes both premolars and molars, or a total of twenty teeth.

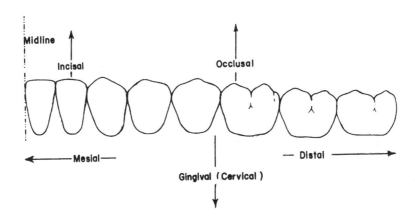

C. Tooth surfaces:

    1. Anteriors - All anterior teeth exhibit four surfaces and one edge on their crowns. They are named as follows:

        a. Mesial - The surface toward the midline.

        b. Distal - The surface away from the midline.

        c. Labial -The "outside" surface which is toward the lips.

        d. Lingual - The "inside" surface which is toward the tongue. In the maxillary arch, the lingual surface is sometimes called the palatal surface.

        e. Incisal edge (or ridge) - The biting edge.

    2. Posteriors - All posterior teeth exhibit five surfaces on their crowns:

        a. Mesial, distal, and lingual - These surfaces may be defined like the corresponding surfaces of anterior teeth.

        b. Buccal - The "outside" surface which is toward the cheek, and corresponds to the labial surface of the anterior teeth. The term facial surface may be used for either the labial surface of anterior teeth or the buccal surface of posterior teeth.

        c. Occlusal - The chewing surface.

    3. Roots - Root surfaces are named exactly like the surfaces of crowns, except there is no incisal edge or occlusal surface. The termination or tip of the root is termed the apex (Plural - apices).

    4. Proximal - This term refers to any surface between two teeth, so proximal surfaces, by definition, are normally only mesial or distal surfaces.

13

SURFACES

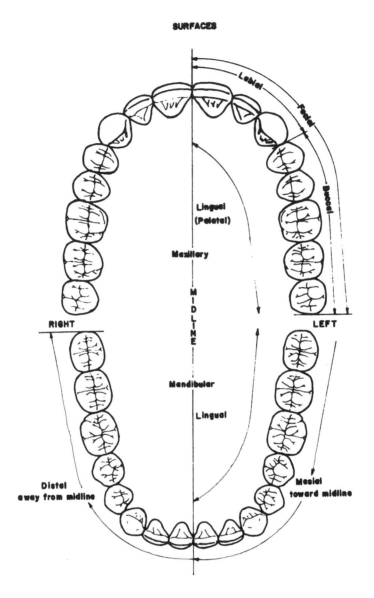

D. <u>Line angle</u> - The line, or angle formed by the junction of two crown surfaces, and its name is derived by combining the names of those two surfaces.

When naming line angles and point angles, the names of the surfaces are combined by dropping the "al" from the end of the first surface and substituting an "o." Where two "o's" are adjacent, they are separated by a hyphen.

There are thus eight line angles on each tooth, and they are listed as follows:

1. Line angles of anterior teeth:

mesiolabial	labioincisal
mesiolingual	linguoincisal
distolabial	mesioincisal
distolingual	distoincisal

14

2. Line angles of posterior teeth:

mesiobuccal	bucco-occlusal
mesiolingual	linguo-occlusal
distobuccal	disto-occlusal
distolingual	mesio-occlusal

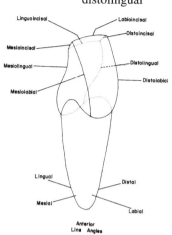

Anterior
Line Angles

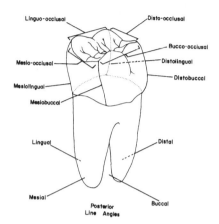

Posterior
Line Angles

E. <u>Point angle</u> - The point which is the junction of three crown surfaces, and takes the name of those three surfaces.

1. Point angles of anterior teeth:

mesiolabioincisal
mesiolinguoincisal
distolabioincisal
distolinguoincisal

2. Point angles of posterior teeth:

mesiobucco-occlusal
mesiolinguo-occlusal
distobucco-occlusal
distolinguo-occlusal

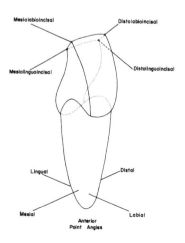

Anterior
Point Angles

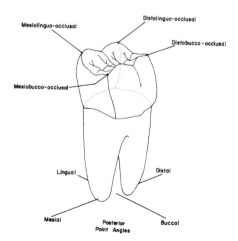

Posterior
Point Angles

15

F. Thirds of crown and root:

1. Crown - The crown surfaces of teeth are divided into artificial thirds, both horizontally and vertically. These thirds are named by their location, according to the surface which is being viewed. For example, the mesial crown surface of an anterior tooth exhibits labial, middle and lingual thirds, when divided vertically. When divided horizontally, this same mesial crown surface has incisal, middle, and cervical thirds.

2. Root - The root, from any aspect, is divided into horizontal thirds only, which are termed cervical, middle, and apical thirds. The term "cervical" denotes toward the cervix, or neck of the tooth, or in other words, toward the cervical line. The cervical thirds of the root and crown are thus adjacent to each other and are separated by the cervical line.

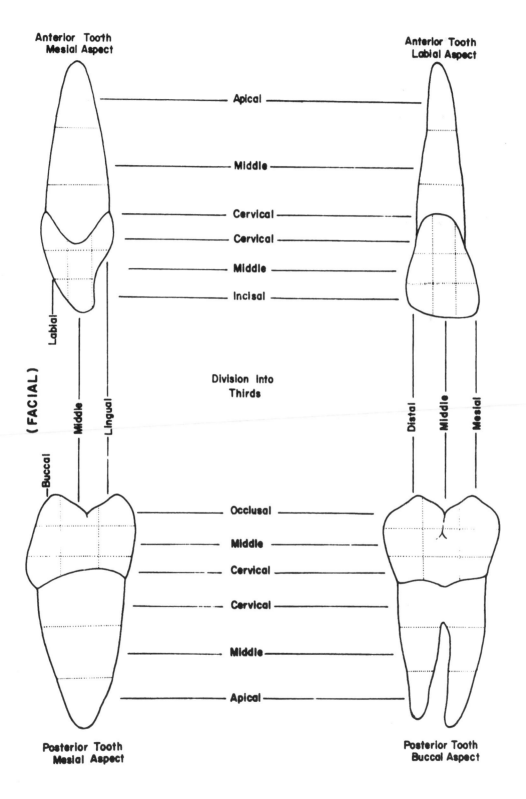

Anterior Tooth
Mesial Aspect

Anterior Tooth
Labial Aspect

Apical

Middle

Cervical

Cervical

Middle

Incisal

Labial

Middle

Lingual

(FACIAL)

Division Into
Thirds

Distal

Middle

Mesial

Buccal

Occlusal

Middle

Cervical

Cervical

Middle

Apical

Posterior Tooth
Mesial Aspect

Posterior Tooth
Buccal Aspect

17

X. Other Anatomical Structures Defined:

A. Crown Elevations:

1. <u>Cusps</u> - Elevated and usually pointed projections of various sizes and shapes on the crowns of teeth. They form the bulk of the occlusal surfaces of posterior teeth, and the incisal portion of canine crowns. Incisors do not possess cusps, while canines normally exhibit one cusp, premolars two or three cusps, and molars usually four or more.

2. <u>Tubercles</u> - Rounded or pointed projections found on the crowns of teeth. Tubercles are not a normal finding, although they are not rare. They are also variable in size and shape, but are usually smaller than cusps. Tubercles are often thought of as minicusps, and their most likely location is on the lingual surface of maxillary anterior teeth, especially deciduous canines. The <u>Cusp of Carabelli</u>, a tubercle, is a normal finding on the mesial part of the lingual surface of permanent maxillary first molars.

3. <u>Cingulum</u> (Plural - cingula) - A large rounded eminence on the lingual surface of all permanent and deciduous anterior teeth, which encompasses the entire cervical third of the lingual surface.

4. Ridges - Linear and usually convex elevations on the surfaces of the crowns of teeth, which are named according to their location. Several specific types of ridges can be identified as follows:

   a. <u>Marginal ridges</u> - The linear elevations which are convex in cross section and are found at the mesial and distal terminations of the occlusal surface of posterior teeth. They are also found on anterior teeth, but are less prominent. Their location also differs, since on anterior teeth they form the lateral (mesial and distal) margins of the lingual surface.

   b. <u>Triangular ridges</u> - Linear ridges which descend from the tips of cusps of posterior teeth toward the central area of the occlusal surface. In cross-section, they are more or less triangular, hence their name.

   c. <u>Transverse ridge</u> - The combination of two triangular ridges, which transversely cross the occlusal surface on a posterior tooth to merge with each other. Thus a transverse ridge is simply a union of two triangular ridges of a posterior tooth, one from a buccal cusp and the other from a lingual cusp and also is composed of two triangular ridges.

   d. <u>Oblique ridge</u> - A special type of transverse ridge, which crosses the occlusal surface of most maxillary molars of both dentitions in an oblique direction from the distobuccal to mesiolingual cusps.

   e. <u>Cusp ridges</u> - Each cusp has four cusp ridges extending in different directions (mesial, distal, facial, lingual) from its tip. They vary in size, shape, and sharpness. Normally, the cusp ridge which extends toward the central portion   of the occlusal surface is also a triangular ridge. They are named by the direction they extend from the cusp tip.

   f. <u>Inclined plane</u> - The sloping area found between two cusp ridges. Planes are named by combining the names of the two cusp ridges between which they lie. Normally, each cusp exhibits four inclined planes.

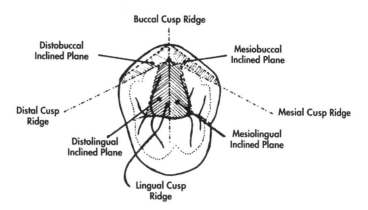

Buccal Cusp Ridge

Distobuccal Inclined Plane

Mesiobuccal Inclined Plane

Distal Cusp Ridge

Mesial Cusp Ridge

Distolingual Inclined Plane

Mesiolingual Inclined Plane

Lingual Cusp Ridge

5. <u>Mamelons</u> - Small, rounded projections of enamel which are found in varying sizes and numbers on the incisal ridges of recently erupted incisors. They
are normally worn away rather soon after eruption, if the tooth contacts its
antagonist(s) in the opposite arch when in function.

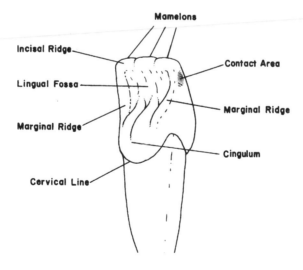

Mamelons

Incisal Ridge

Contact Area

Lingual Fossa

Marginal Ridge

Marginal Ridge

Cingulum

Cervical Line

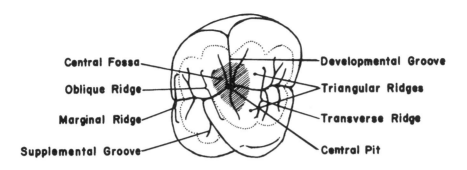

Central Fossa — Developmental Groove
Oblique Ridge — Triangular Ridges
Marginal Ridge — Transverse Ridge
Supplemental Groove — Central Pit

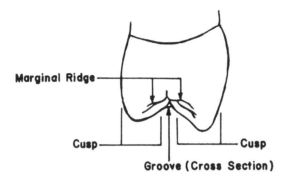

Marginal Ridge

Cusp — Cusp

Groove (Cross Section)

B.   Crown Depressions:

1.   <u>Fossa</u> (Plural - fossae) - An irregular, usually rounded depression, or concavity, on the crown of a tooth. There is normally a rather large, shallow fossa
on the lingual surface of anterior teeth, while posterior teeth exhibit two or
more fossae of varying size and shape on the occlusal surface.

2.   <u>Developmental (primary) groove</u> - A groove, or line, which usually denotes the coalescence of the primary parts, or lobes, of the crown of a tooth.

3.   <u>Supplemental (secondary) groove</u> - An auxiliary groove which branches
from a developmental groove. Its location is not related to the junction of primary tooth parts, and it is normally not as deep as a primary groove.

4.   <u>Pit</u> - A small, depressed area where developmental grooves often join or
terminate. A pit is usually found in the deepest portion of a fossa.

C.   Miscellaneous Structures:

1.   <u>Contact area</u> - The area on a proximal surface of the crown that contacts the
adjacent tooth in the same arch, and is thus named mesial or distal by location.
All teeth in each quadrant normally have two contact areas, except the most
distal tooth which, of course, has no distal contact area.

2.   <u>Lobe</u> - One of the primary anatomical divisions of the tooth crown, often
separated by identifiable developmental grooves.

UNIT # 2

I. **Reading Assignment:**

Unit # 2 (Anatomic and Physiologic Considerations of Form and Function)

II. **Specific Objectives:**

At the completion of this unit, the student will be able to:

A. Differentiate between the following terms by correctly defining, or by selecting the proper response from a series of definitions or their applications.

1. Periodontium
2. Lobe
3. Curve of Spee
4. Curve of Wilson
5. Compensating occlusal curvature
6. Axial position
7. Contact area
8. Interproximal space
9. Embrasure
10. Line angle
11. Height of contour
12. Cervical line
13. Gingival line
14. Epithelial attachment

B. Name the three major functions of the human dentition, or select the correct response from a series of choices which relate to these functions or their applications.

C. Select the correct response from a series of choices which describe the steps involved in the evolution of the human dental mechanism, or how these steps relate to form and function.

D. Provide an understanding of lobes by correctly selecting from a series of choices, or identifying from a two-dimensional diagram, the number and names of the lobes of the anterior and posterior teeth, the major portions of each tooth which compose lobes, and the major structures separating lobes.

E. Differentiate between the general axial positions of any of the various permanent teeth, by selecting the correct response from a series of descriptions or diagrams.

F. Differentiate between the crown surfaces of teeth by matching them with their correct general shape (triangular, trapezoidal, or rhomboidal), or by relating the shape to the specific function of the tooth.

G. Describe, or differentiate between contact areas by providing, or selecting from a series of choices the correct information which relates to the:

1. two purposes served by proper contact areas.
2. general rules of size and location on individual teeth.
3. differences between the contact areas of anterior and posterior teeth.
4. changes in contact areas occurring with age.

H. Describe, or correctly select from a series of choices, the components, boundaries, or functions of the interproximal space.

I.   Describe, or differentiate between embrasures by providing, or selecting from a series of choices, the correct:

1.   information regarding the two purposes embrasures serve.

2.   information regarding the general rules of normal embrasure form.

3.   names of embrasures, when given a description or two-dimensional diagram.

J.   Describe, or select from a list of choices the correct information regarding the proper location of the height of contour on the facial and lingual surfaces of the teeth, and its major contribution to gingival health.

K.   Differentiate between the levels, depths, and directions of curvature of the cervical lines on all surfaces of both anterior and posterior teeth, by describing them, or by choosing the correct response from a series of choices.

L.   Describe the proper location and form of marginal ridges and facial line angles, and their relationship to embrasure form, by selecting the correct response from a series of choices. In addition, the student will be able to identify the normal location of central grooves and occlusal anatomy of posterior teeth in the same manner.

M.   Identify, or make applications to the type of root structure necessary for proper function of the different teeth, and the general rules regarding tooth roots and normal number of branches, by selecting the correct response from a series of choices.

N.   Demonstrate a knowledge of the protective functional form of the teeth, by correctly labeling, or choosing between diagrams which illustrate proper and improper form, or by matching specific tooth form with its complementary physiologic activity.

The student is also responsible for any material that was to have been mastered in the previous unit.

UNIT # 2
ANATOMIC AND PHYSIOLOGIC CONSIDERATIONS
OF FORM AND FUNCTION

I. **Introduction:**

A. Almost all entities in nature display a form which can be intimately related to their purpose and function. Teeth are no exception, and the forms which human teeth exhibit are an evolutionary product to best fulfill their specific functions. This is not only true of natural systems, but also of most man-made materials. For example, if one notes the form of various dental instruments, he soon realizes that each instrument has a specific form to accomplish a specific function in the most efficient manner.

B. The three major functions of human teeth, to which their general form, contours, and alignment are directly related, are:

    1. <u>Mastication</u> - chewing.

    2. <u>Esthetics</u> - appearance.

    3. <u>Phonetics</u> - speech.

To best accomplish these three functions, the teeth display certain forms which align and stabilize the entire dentition, and protect the teeth and their associated structures from insult and potential deterioration. Even one aberrant tooth contour may lead to the breakdown of the entire dental mechanism.

C. This unit, then, is devoted to a limited discussion of normal tooth form and alignment as they are related to function. It is intended to form the basis of respect for, and a philosophy of, physiologic considerations of the teeth, and their supporting structures. This philosophy should help harmonize the dentist's procedures with the ideals of preservation and prevention, in contrast to the purely mechanical approach of a "tooth carpenter." The dentist who pays no heed to normal tooth form and alignment, when planning or placing restorations, may well be creating more potential damage to the dental mechanism than can be corrected by the dental procedures.

D. The <u>periodontium</u> is simply the supporting tissues, both hard and soft, of a tooth. It is the periodontium, all, or a portion of which, may suffer the consequences of anomalous natural tooth forms, or dentist-induced (iatrogenic) imperfections.

II. **Comparative Dental Anatomy:**

A. Since man is not the only animal with teeth, an overview of the dental systems of some other animals, past and present, is of value in projecting evolutionary patterns, and making contemporary comparisons. This section will be brief, but the interested student will find in-depth discussions in other anatomical and anthropological writings.

B. Most present day vertebrates possess teeth. The most primitive type of tooth crown is <u>conical</u> in shape, and is composed of a single cone or lobe. This type of tooth was common in primitive vertebrates, and today is exhibited by many of the lower vertebrates, including the reptiles. These animals are homodonts, with similarly shaped teeth differing only in size. Since jaw movement is directly related to tooth form, these animals possess only up and down (or hinge action) jaw movements, because the single conical cusps lock together on closure, not allowing lateral movements. Consequently, the basic purpose of the teeth of these animals was, and is, related to grasping prey and combat, since food is not masticated, but swallowed whole.

C.   In contrast to the lower vertebrates the dental systems of mammals have evolved with much greater diversity. The evolutionary step that made this possible was the development of the <u>tritubercular</u>, or three-lobed (cusped) tooth. From the tritubercular tooth, mammals have evolved additional lobes, so that most mammalian teeth exhibit four or more lobes. Unlike the lower vertebrates, which are generally homodont, mammals exhibit differing tooth forms, and thus are heterodont in nature. Furthermore, mammals are the only animals which may display more than a single root per tooth. A mammal which is fully heterodont, but still lacks lateral jaw movements, due to interlocking cusps, is the dog. This type of hinge axis is common to most other carnivores, as well. In contrast, the bear has a dentition more suited to its omnivorous diet. Although still retaining the elongated incisors and canines (fangs) of the dog, the bear has flattened posterior teeth with enlarged occlusal surfaces. This allows for some lateral jaw movements similar to man, although they are more limited.

D.   The most highly developed and complex teeth, where the crowns are normally composed of four or more lobes, belong to those animals which are members of the order of mammals known as primates. Along with man, this order includes apes and monkeys. Excluding man, most primates exist in a tropical climate, with a basically herbivorous diet of fruits. Some of the primates, for example the anthropoid ape, have dental formulae identical to man. However, these animals have retained elongated canines from an evolutionary past which was carnivorous, and hence do not have quite the latitude of jaw movement found in man.

E.   At the top of the ladder, man has evolved the most complex dental mechanism of all animals. Being omnivorous, homo sapiens has developed teeth to function both in the mastication of meat and plant foods. The elongated and interlocking canines have been reduced in length so that they function with the rest of the teeth in lateral movements, and the individual teeth differ in both size and development from other primates. All teeth in the human dentition are comprised of four or more lobes.

F.   There is one group of mammals which displays a greater range of jaw movement than does man. The hoofed mammals, or ungulates, which include the cow, horse, and deer, exhibit extensive latitude of jaw movement during mastication of their entirely herbivorous diet.

G.   The form to function relationship has evolved some interesting types of teeth to perform functions unique to certain animals. Notable examples include the incisors of most rodents, especially the beaver, and the hollow canine fangs of certain poisonous reptiles.

III.   Lobes:

A.   Introduction:

The previous section pointed out that animal teeth developed evolutionarily from a one-lobed, conical crown, through the tritubercular, or three-lobed form, to the four or more lobed crowns found in the primates. <u>Lobe</u> was defined as a primary division of the tooth in the previous unit. Until recently, it was believed that each lobe developed from a separate calcification center, but this theory has fallen into disfavor in the last few years. Therefore, lobes will be considered only as anatomical divisions of a tooth, often separated by distinguishable primary grooves. The lobe pattern in the human dentition plays a part in the form and function of each individual tooth.

B.   Permanent Anterior Teeth:

All anterior teeth are composed of four lobes. There are three labial lobes, named <u>mesiolabial</u>, <u>middle labial</u>, and <u>distolabial lobes</u>. (Occasionally the middle labial lobe is referred to simply as the <u>labial lobe</u>.) The remaining lobe encompasses the cingulum, and is termed the <u>lingual lobe</u>.

Evidence for the presence of the three labial lobes is sometimes found on the incisal edge of newly erupted incisors in the form of mamelons, which are the slightly rounded incisal terminations of the labial lobes. When the incisors are in functional occlusion, the mamelons are abraded away soon after eruption, but may still be visible, even in adults, when the incisor has not been in active occlusion.

Further evidence of separation of the labial lobes of all anterior teeth is found in the form of two shallow depressions in the incisal portion of the labial surface. These linear, vertical depressions are called mesiolabial and distolabial developmental depressions.

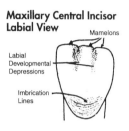

Maxillary Central Incisor
Labial View

Mamelons

Labial Developmental Depressions

Imbrication Lines

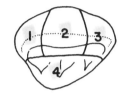

Maxillary Central Incisor
1. Distolabial lobe
2. Middle Labial lobe
3. Mesiolabial lobe
4. Lingual lobe

C. Permanent Posterior Teeth:

1. Premolars - Most premolars also exhibit four lobes, three buccal and one lingual. They are named mesiobuccal, middle buccal, distobuccal, and lingual lobes. The one exception is the mandibular second premolar which, in the majority of cases, exhibits two lingual cusps. When this is the case, there are five lobes, three on the buccal and two lingually located. The three buccal lobes are named as in the four-lobed type, while the lingual lobes are termed mesiolingual and distolingual lobes.

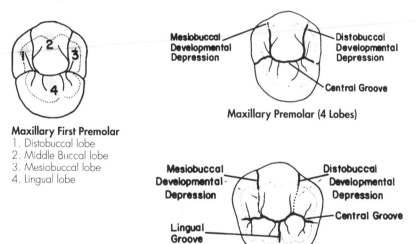

Maxillary First Premolar
1. Distobuccal lobe
2. Middle Buccal lobe
3. Mesiobuccal lobe
4. Lingual lobe

Mesiobuccal Developmental Depression

Distobuccal Developmental Depression

Central Groove

Maxillary Premolar (4 Lobes)

Mesiobuccal Developmental Depression

Distobuccal Developmental Depression

Central Groove

Lingual Groove

Mandibular Second Premolar (5 Lobes)

As with the labial surface of the anterior teeth, the buccal surface of premolars normally displays lobe division in the form of mesiobuccal and distobuccal developmental depressions. When viewed from the occlusal aspect, the central groove serves as the separation between the buccal lobes and the lingual lobe(s). In the case of the mandibular second premolar with two lingual cusps, the lingual groove separates the two lingual lobes.

2. Permanent Molars:

a. Maxillary Molars - Normally, maxillary molars have four lobes, two buccal and two lingual, which are named in the same manner as the cusps that represent them (<u>mesiobuccal</u>, <u>distobuccal</u>, <u>mesiolingual</u>, and <u>distolingual lobes</u>). Unlike the anterior teeth and premolars, molars do not exhibit facial developmental depressions. Evidence of lobe separation can be found in the central groove, which divides buccal from lingual lobes. The two lingual lobes are separated by the distolingual groove, and the two buccal lobes are divided by the buccal groove.

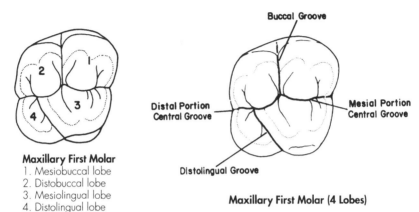

Maxillary First Molar
1. Mesiobuccal lobe
2. Distobuccal lobe
3. Mesiolingual lobe
4. Distolingual lobe

Maxillary First Molar (4 Lobes)

b. Mandibular first molars - These teeth normally have five cusps and five lobes. They are named for the cusps, exactly like the lobes of maxillary molars, with the addition of the fifth lobe, the <u>distal lobe</u>. Separational evidence is found in the central groove, as well as the lingual groove, buccal groove, and distobuccal groove.

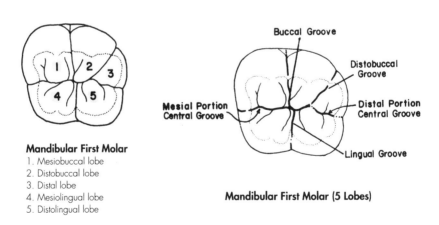

Mandibular First Molar
1. Mesiobuccal lobe
2. Distobuccal lobe
3. Distal lobe
4. Mesiolingual lobe
5. Distolingual lobe

Mandibular First Molar (5 Lobes)

c. Other mandibular molars - The crowns of most other mandibular molars exhibit four cusps and four lobes, with terminology the same as it is for maxillary molars. The developmental grooves indicative of lobe division include the central, buccal, and lingual grooves.

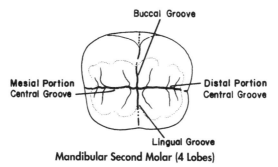

Buccal Groove

Mesial Portion
Central Groove

Distal Portion
Central Groove

Lingual Groove

Mandibular Second Molar (4 Lobes)

IV. General Occlusal Curvatures and Axial Position:

A. The general arrangement of the arches and the inclinations of the individual teeth are interrelated in such a manner as to allow the most efficient use of the forces of mastication, while at the same time stabilizing and protecting the dental arches.

B. <u>Curve of Spee</u> - The curvature which begins at the tip of the canines and follows the buccal cusp tips of the premolars and molars posteriorly, when viewed from their facial aspect. The Curve of Spee is two dimensional, and curves upward from anterior to posterior. It can readily be seen how the inclination of some of the individual posterior teeth must be offset from the vertical long axis of the body, if their occlusal surfaces are to conform to this curve. Maxillary molar roots are inclined mesially and mandibular molar roots distally.

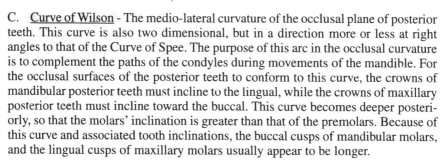

CURVE OF SPEE

C. <u>Curve of Wilson</u> - The medio-lateral curvature of the occlusal plane of posterior teeth. This curve is also two dimensional, but in a direction more or less at right angles to that of the Curve of Spee. The purpose of this arc in the occlusal curvature is to complement the paths of the condyles during movements of the mandible. For the occlusal surfaces of the posterior teeth to conform to this curve, the crowns of mandibular posterior teeth must incline to the lingual, while the crowns of maxillary posterior teeth must incline toward the buccal. This curve becomes deeper posteriorly, so that the molars' inclination is greater than that of the premolars. Because of this curve and associated tooth inclinations, the buccal cusps of mandibular molars, and the lingual cusps of maxillary molars usually appear to be longer.

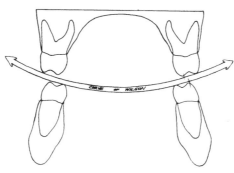

CURVE OF WILSON

D. <u>Compensating Occlusal Curvature</u> (Sphere of Monson) - The three dimensional curvature of the occlusal plane, which is the combination of the Curve of Spee and the Curve of Wilson. From this definition, it can be seen that this curvature is in the form of a portion of a ball, or sphere. Therefore, this curvature is concave for the mandibular arch and convex for the maxillary arch.

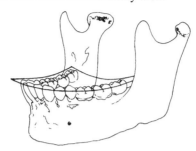

E. <u>Axial Position</u> - The inclination of a tooth from a vertical axis. This inclination is normally described in mesiodistal and faciolingual directions, even though it is usually an inseparable combination of the two. Further, it is normally described in terms of the root's inclination, which means that the crown is normally inclined in the opposite direction. These inclinations are necessary for proper occlusal and incisal function of the teeth. There is a wide range of axial positions, as is evident from the following descriptions for individual permanent teeth. As these axial positions are described, it should be of value to relate them to the individual tooth's functions, as well as its inclination relative to the Curves of Spee and Wilson.

1. Maxillary anterior teeth: The maxillary anterior teeth exhibit great inclination of the root toward the lingual, when considering the faciolingual dimension. In the mesiodistal direction, the maxillary incisors' roots incline very slightly toward the mesial, but the canine root inclines toward the distal.

2. Maxillary premolars: Maxillary premolars' root inclinations are slight: toward the lingual in the faciolingual dimension, and toward the distal in the mesiodistal dimension.

3. Maxillary molars: The roots of maxillary molars display great lingual inclination, and moderate mesial inclination.

4. Mandibular anterior teeth: The mandibular incisors and canines exhibit great lingual root inclinations in the faciolingual direction. Mesiodistally, the incisors are nearly straight, or display only minor mesial root inclination, while the canines have slight distal root inclination.

5. Mandibular premolars: Mesiodistally, these teeth show some distal root inclination. An interesting situation occurs in the faciolingual direction, since the first premolar's root inclines lingually, but the second premolar's root is offset buccally, both inclinations being slight.

6. Mandibular molars: The mandibular molars exhibit moderate to great buccal and distal root angulations.

V. Crown Surface Form:

A. Introduction:

The geometric configuration of all the crown surfaces of teeth (except incisal and occlusal) can be placed in one of three general categories: <u>triangular</u>, <u>trapezoidal</u>, or <u>rhomboidal</u>.

B.   Facial and Lingual Surfaces:

From the facial and lingual aspects, all permanent teeth in the mouth can be roughly described as <u>trapezoidal.</u> The incisal (occlusal) side forms the base of the trapezoid, while the cervical represents the shorter parallel side. Arrangement of these trapezoidal shaped crowns side by side in the dental arches creates <u>interproximal spaces</u> between the teeth, as well as one <u>contact area</u> between each pair of adjacent teeth. Since the shorter parallel side of the trapezoid is at the cervical, there is adequate space available for bony support around the roots of each tooth.

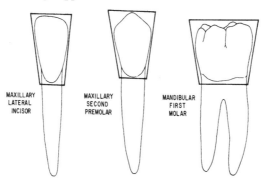

MAXILLARY LATERAL INCISOR   MAXILLARY SECOND PREMOLAR   MANDIBULAR FIRST MOLAR

C.   Mesial and Distal Surfaces:

1.   Anterior teeth: As viewed from their proximal surfaces, the crowns of permanent anterior teeth exhibit a <u>triangular</u> shape, with the base of the triangle at the cervical, and the apex at the incisal. This shape readily fits into the prescribed function of the anterior teeth, since the apex at the incisal functions as a wedge in tearing, biting, and incising food material, while the wider cervical base provides the necessary strength for the crown form.

2.   Maxillary posterior teeth: The crowns of permanent maxillary posterior teeth have proximal surfaces which are roughly <u>trapezoidal</u> in shape, with the base at the cervical, and buccal and lingual sides constricting toward the occlusal. This general shape also provides a wedge form which aids in the distribution of forces during mastication, and facilitates the self-cleaning process of the teeth.

3.   Mandibular posterior teeth: From the proximal aspect, permanent mandibular posterior teeth are roughly <u>rhomboidal,</u> with the crowns inclined toward the lingual. This form and inclination allows for proper interlocking of the mandibular and maxillary posterior teeth during mastication.

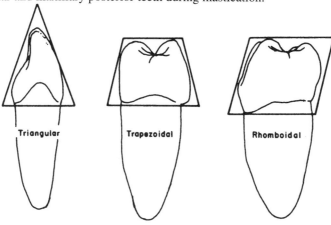

Triangular   Trapezoidal   Rhomboidal

VI.   Contact Areas:

A.   In a complete arch, each tooth touches or contacts two adjacent teeth, with the exception of the most posterior tooth in the arch, which has only a tooth to its mesial to contact. The places where the teeth do touch are called <u>contact areas</u>. These proximal contact areas are normally between the mesial surface of one tooth and the distal surface of the tooth just anterior to it, except where the central incisors contact each other at the midline, and then mesial surface contacts mesial surface.

B.   Normally, contact areas increase in size with age. Shortly after eruption and initial contact with adjacent teeth, they approach a "point" in size, but with age they broaden and may rightfully be called a contact "area". This broadening is due to the abrasion that occurs when the proximal surfaces of the teeth rub against each other. As a result of this abrasive action, the mesiodistal length of the dental arches continuously becomes shorter. This is a slow but dynamic process; as the teeth become narrower mesiodistally, they are actually moving mesially, or closer to the midline.

C.   The proper location of contact areas aids in stabilizing the dental arch. Another function which proper contact areas serve is the prevention of food material from slipping between the teeth. The chronic packing of food usually results in an inflammation of the supporting soft tissues, which in turn may lead to a breakdown of the bony component of the periodontium. Thus, the replacement of a proper contact area in dental restorations is of extreme importance.

D.   Not only must the contact area be tight to prevent food packing, but its proper location, both in an inciso (occluso) cervical direction and a faciolingual direction, is also important in the food flow pattern.

E.   The normal location of the contact areas for individual permanent teeth will be discussed in the succeeding units, so only the following general rules will be presented here:

1.   Contact areas become more cervically located from anterior to posterior in each quadrant.

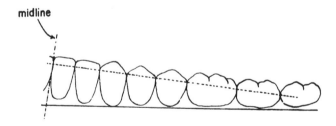

2.   On an individual tooth, the distal contact area normally has a more cervical location than the mesial contact area.

3.   The relative size of the contact areas increases from anterior to posterior in each quadrant.

4.   Anterior teeth have contact areas which are normally centered in the faciolingual dimension.

5.   Posterior teeth have contact areas which are normally located to the buccal of center in the faciolingual dimension.

VII. Interproximal Spaces:

A. The <u>interproximal space</u> is the triangular shaped area between adjacent teeth in the same arch cervical to the contact area, and which is best observed from the facial aspect. Usually, the interproximal space is filled with that portion of the periodontium known as the <u>gingival tissue</u>, or more specifically, as the <u>interdental papilla</u>. The triangle is formed by alveolar bone at its cervical base, the proximal surfaces of the adjacent teeth on its sides, and the contact area of the adjacent teeth at its apex. These structures are thus the boundaries of the interproximal space.

B. The size and shape of the interproximal space depend on the form and location of all its boundaries. The general triangular shape is of consequence to the health of the entire periodontium, and is especially important to the proper stimulation of the periodontium. This shape also aids in the self-cleaning process of the dentition.

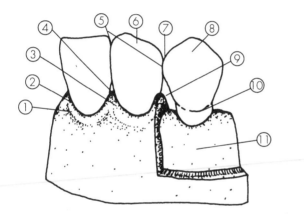

1. Marginal Gingiva
2. Gingival Line
3. Interdental Papilla
4. Gingival Embrasure
5. Contact Area
6. Clinical Crown
7. Incisal/Occlusal Embrasure
8. Anatomical Crown
9. Interproximal Space
10. Cervical Line (CEJ)
11. Alveolar Bone

INTERPROXIMAL SPACE AND
RELATED STRUCTURES

VIII. Embrasures:

A. <u>Embrasure</u> - The open space between the proximal surfaces of two adjacent teeth in the same arch, where they diverge facially or lingually, and incisally (occlusally) or cervically from the contact area.

B. Embrasures are named according to their location, which depends on the aspect from which the teeth are being viewed. When viewing the teeth from either the facial or lingual aspects, the two embrasures which may be observed are the <u>incisal (occlusal)</u> and <u>cervical (gingival) embrasures</u>. The cervical embrasure corresponds to the interproximal space, and is normally larger in area than the incisal (occlusal) embrasure.

When viewing the teeth from the incisal or occlusal aspect, the two embrasures which are visible are named <u>labial (buccal)</u> and <u>lingual embrasures</u>.

C.   Ideally, if an imaginary line is drawn to bisect any embrasure space, the two portions so described should be approximately equal in size and shape, or in other words they should be symmetrical. This is extremely important when planning or performing dental operations, for if one side of the embrasure is contoured differently than the other, it may affect the health of the periodontium. For example, if the dentist finds that the outline of one of the adjacent teeth is slightly convex, the restoration placed on the other tooth should also be slightly convex in this area. In addition, asymmetrical embrasure form in the anterior teeth may compromise esthetics.

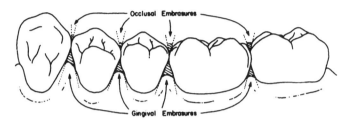

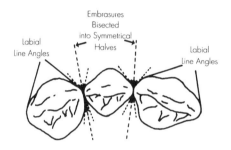

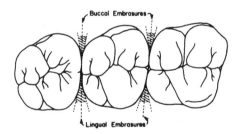

D.   Proper embrasure form has two main physiological purposes:

1.   To serve as a spillway for the food material during mastication.

2.   To serve as an integral part of the self-cleaning process of the teeth.

These two purposes are interrelated, and tend to complement each other in both the protection and stimulation of the periodontium. Improper embrasure form may result in a lack of protection, with resultant overstimulation of the periodontium, and its potential breakdown. Overprotection, with a resultant lack of stimulation of the periodontium, also may result in its breakdown.

In the anterior part of the mouth, embrasure form is also a factor in the esthetics function of the human dentition.

E. Some general rules regarding normal embrasure form are as follows:

1. From the facial or lingual aspect, incisal (occlusal) embrasures increase in relative size from the anterior teeth toward the posterior.

2. From the facial or lingual aspect, cervical (gingival) embrasures decrease in relative size from anterior to posterior.

3. From the incisal aspect, the labial and lingual embrasures are nearly equal in size in anterior teeth.

4. From the occlusal aspect, the lingual embrasure is normally larger than the buccal embrasure in posterior teeth.

5. When one side of an embrasure (tooth outline) has a certain contour, the other side of the embrasure will normally have a similar contour.

F. It should now be easy to recognize the interrelation between contact areas and embrasure form. For example, as the contact area becomes more cervically located the farther posteriorly in the arch, the relative size of the incisal (occlusal) embrasure increases, while the relative size of the cervical embrasure decreases. And, as the contact area moves farther to the buccal in the posterior teeth, the lingual embrasure becomes relatively larger.

IX. Facial Line Angles:

A. Line angles were previously defined as the line or angle created by the junction of two crown surfaces of a tooth. The two facial line angles of the anterior teeth and premolars of both arches are normally quite prominent, when compared to the more rounded lingual line angles of the same teeth. Their outline is especially noticeable from the incisal (occlusal) aspect, because they are seen in cross section.

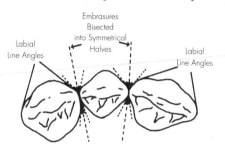

B. These prominent line angles are actually the facial termination of the facial embrasures. For any specific facial embrasure, they are normally located directly adjacent to each other in the faciolingual dimension. For example, the mesiolabial line angle of a lateral incisor should be located directly adjacent (not farther labially or lingually) to the distolabial line angle of the adjacent central incisor. This placement is consistent with the concept of symmetry in embrasure form discussed previously.

X. Facial and Lingual Heights of Contour:

A. Another integral part of the master plan of tooth form and arrangement is the location of the height of contour on the facial and lingual surfaces on the crowns of teeth. The height of contour, which is also known as the crest of curvature, is the greatest area of contour inciso(occluso) cervically on the facial and lingual surfaces, and is best observed by viewing these surface outlines from a proximal aspect. Actually, mesial and distal surfaces also have heights of contour, and they are normally located at the contact areas.

B.   The importance of these contours to the physiology and state of health of the periodontium is also critical. As with embrasure form, these contours aid in the proper protection and stimulation of the gingival tissue. If the contour is excessive, the flow of food material will be deflected away from the gingiva, and inadequate stimulation of these tissues may result in their breakdown. On the other hand, when an insufficient contour does not provide adequate protection, the overstimulation or insult to the gingival tissues may also result in their deterioration. Once again, the implications to the dentist of restoring correct contours should be obvious.

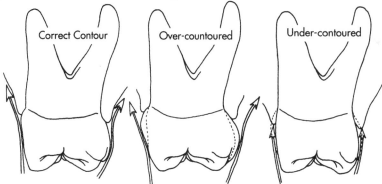

C.   Some general rules concerning the location of heights of contour on the facial and lingual surfaces of the teeth are as follows:

1.   Facial surfaces - The height of contour on the facial surfaces of all anterior and posterior teeth is located in the cervical third.

2.   Lingual surfaces:

a. Anterior teeth - On the lingual surface of incisors and canines, the height of contour is found in the cervical third.

b. Posterior teeth - The lingual height of contour for premolars and molars is located in the middle or occlusal third.

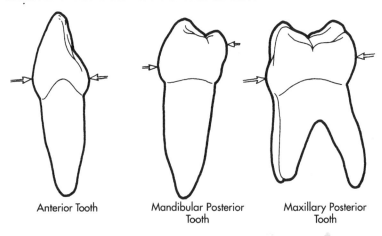

Anterior Tooth   Mandibular Posterior   Maxillary Posterior
                              Tooth   Tooth

XI. Cervical Line Curvatures:

A. Introduction and comparison of terms:.

1. In the preceding unit, the <u>cervical line</u>, or <u>cemento-enamel junction</u>, was defined as the line around the tooth where the enamel and the cementum meet. It is a stable entity, in contrast to the gingival line, which may be ever changing.

2. The <u>gingival line</u>, also called the <u>gingival margin</u> or <u>gingival crest</u>, is the imaginary line which marks the level of termination of the nonattached soft tissue surrounding the tooth. The gingival line level is variable, and usually is above the cervical line early in life, often receding to a lower level as the individual becomes older. The gingival line separates the clinical crown and root, whereas the cervical line separates the anatomical crown and root. The gingival line is always observable clinically, while the cervical line is observable only when not covered by soft tissue, which is in a limited number of teeth.

3. The <u>epithelial attachment</u> is the actual attachment of the soft tissue of the mouth to the tooth. The epithelial attachment can be distinguished from the previously described periodontal ligament even though both structures are components of the tooth's attachment apparatus. The epithelial attachment serves as the connection for the soft (gingival) tissue and is limited in comparative area (but not importance), while the periodontal ligament provides the attachment of the hard tissue (bone) to the tooth's root structure, and is much more extensive in area. Since there is usually a sulcus between the gingival margin and the epithelial attachment, these two entities are not normally located at the same level on the tooth. However, like the gingival margin, the epithelial attachment may be variable in its location, and has a tendency to migrate apically during a person's lifetime, especially in the presence of periodontal disease. The epithelial attachment is normally found close to the level of the CEJ. However, as has been pointed out, the epithelial attachment has a tendency to move apically, so that it is possible for it to be located on the enamel of the cervical third of the crown in young persons, but on the cementum of the root in older individuals.

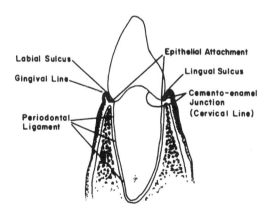

4. On any individual tooth, the amount (depth) of curvature of the cervical line seems to be related to the widths and lengths of the crown, as well as the location of the contact areas proximally.

B. Some general rules concerning cervical line contours in normal dentitions are as follows:

    1. The cervical line is normally curved (convex) or bulges toward the apical on the facial and lingual surfaces of teeth.

    2. The cervical line is normally curved (convex) toward the incisal (occlusal) on the mesial and distal surfaces of teeth.

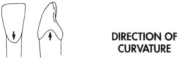

DIRECTION OF CURVATURE

    3. The amount (depth) of cervical line curvature on any individual tooth is normally greater on the mesial, as compared to the distal surface.

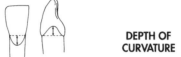

DEPTH OF CURVATURE

    4. Cervical lines on adjacent proximal surfaces of adjacent teeth have approximately the same depth of curvature.

    5. The depth of the curvature on all surfaces is greatest on central incisors, and decreases posteriorly.

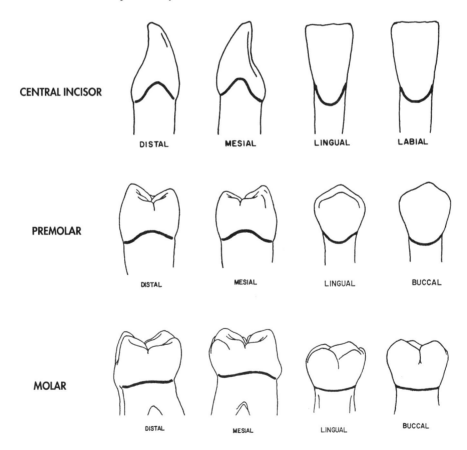

36

XII. Continuity of Marginal Ridges:

A.   In the preceding unit, the term, <u>marginal ridge</u>, was defined. It was pointed out that marginal ridges are the mesial and distal terminations of the occlusal surfaces of posterior teeth, and the lingual surfaces of anterior teeth. Furthermore, it was noted that they are normally bulkier on posterior teeth.

B.   The importance of marginal ridges to the form and function theme of this unit relates partially to their height. The height of the marginal ridges of adjacent teeth in the same arch should be at the same level. In the mouth, this is normally true, unless the teeth are malposed, or one or more missing teeth in the dentition has allowed tipping, supraeruption, or rotation of any of the remaining teeth.

C.   In conjunction with their heights, adjacent marginal ridges are normally shaped so that they create a small occlusal embrasure for posterior teeth or lingual embrasure for anterior teeth. The heights and shapes of the adjacent marginal ridges directly affect the embrasure form. Since the purposes of proper embrasure form have already been discussed, it should be sufficient to remind the reader of the dentist's responsibility to symmetrical embrasure form by establishing marginal ridges on adjacent teeth which are similar in height and shape.

XIII. Continuity of Central Grooves of Posterior Teeth:

The central developmental grooves of posterior teeth are normally aligned into one, more or less continuous valley in each quadrant. This allows for a trough antero-posteriorly through the centers of the occlusal surfaces of the posterior teeth, which results in a more efficient food flow pattern during mastication.

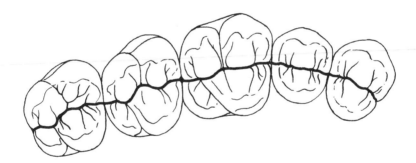

XIV. Occlusal Anatomy:

Another feature of posterior teeth is the groove and ridge pattern on the masticating surface, or in other words, the <u>occlusal anatomy</u>. Since a future occlusion course will describe how occlusal anatomy is related to function, only a general statement will be made: In any dental restorative procedure, the occlusal anatomy of a tooth should normally be reproduced to preexisting form, location, and relative height or depth.

XV. Root Shape and Number of Branches:

A. The shape, length, and number of root branches are also intimately related to a tooth's form and function. The canine, by virtue of its location in the arch, and its evolutionary function as the fang of carnivores, has the longest and strongest root in both arches. The molars are multirooted to complement the increased size of the occlusal table, as they function in grinding. And so it is with all tooth roots; their form is directly related to crown form, placement in the arch, and function.

B. Some general rules regarding tooth roots and branches are as follows:

1. Roots are normally widest toward the cervical area and taper toward the apex.

2. Anterior teeth and premolars normally have single roots. An exception is the maxillary first premolar, which normally exhibits two root branches, a buccal and a lingual.

3. Maxillary molars normally possess three roots, one lingual and two buccal branches.

4. Mandibular molars normally have two roots, one mesial and one distal branch.

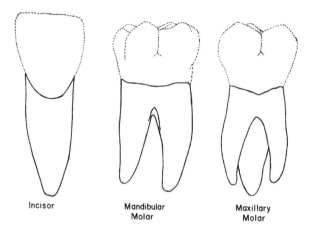

Incisor   Mandibular Molar   Maxillary Molar

XVI. Conclusion:

A. At this point, the reader should be cognizant of two points which have been emphasized throughout this unit:

1. Tooth form and function are directly related.

2. The potential for the breakdown of the periodontium is directly related to form and function, and the dentist is under an obligation to understand and apply the principles of form and function in all dental procedures.

B. With the first two units as background, the student should now be prepared to study the individual permanent teeth in detail. During study of the remaining text, the student should make use of the principles of this unit in understanding why certain structures take certain forms, and why they are located where they are.

INTRODUCTION TO THE STUDY OF
INDIVIDUAL PERMANENT TEETH

The succeeding six units describe the permanent teeth in detail. There are several suggestions that may be of value during the study of these units:

1. In the first two units, a number of general rules were presented. Remember that these are only "general" rules, and they will occasionally reflect exceptions and discrepancies as the permanent teeth are studied in detail.

2. Always keep in mind that the text's description of an individual tooth is really a composite or "average" representation, and that natural teeth may vary widely in their morphology and anatomy. Therefore, it is not realistic to expect every tooth in the mouth to appear as a carbon copy of its counterpart in the text.

3. One point in the preface is worth reemphasizing, and that is the use of the diagrams and models in conjunction with the written descriptions.

4. For the sake of brevity, usually only the first tooth of a series is described in complete detail. Thereafter, similarities in any of the succeeding teeth are usually omitted and only differences are described. Therefore, any apparent omissions should be regarded as similarities to the initial tooth in the series. For example, in Unit # 3, the central incisors are described in great detail, but the sections covering the lateral incisors are much briefer.

5. During the description of tooth surfaces, the terms "margin" and "outline" are synonymous. For example: "The mesial margin/outline of the buccal surface is . . . . "

6. The terms "height of contour" and "crest of curvature" are also synonymous. Keep in mind, however, that the height of contour or crest of curvature may be differently located for the surface as a whole, than it is for a margin or outline of that surface. For example: The height of contour of the facial surface of a certain tooth will be located in the cervical third, whereas the height of contour for the distal outline of the facial surface might be located in the occlusal third.

7. In these units, there is a section entitled "variations and anomalies" associated with each permanent tooth. In reality, anomalies are abnormalities, or a departure from regular conditions, whereas extremes in morphology which fit into a range of variation in size and shape, etc., are not considered anomalous. However, both true anomalies and extremes in the range of variations will be considered in these sections.

8. To place the content of these units into proper perspective, just look into the future when you will be performing dental procedures in a patient's mouth, and attempt to visualize the effect on these procedures of being able to recognize both the normal and abnormal morphology of individual teeth.

UNIT # 3

I. **Reading Assignment:**

Introduction to the Study of Individual Permanent Teeth & Unit # 3 (The Permanent Incisors)

II. **Specific Objectives:**

At the completion of this unit, the student will be able to:

A. List the appropriate age(s) concerning developmental chronology of the permanent incisors found in the development tables, or select the appropriate age(s) from a list, when given a certain developmental feature. The student should also be able to compare these ages among the permanent incisors.

B. Demonstrate a knowledge of the morphology of each surface of the crown, as well as the root, of each permanent incisor by:

1. describing,

2. selecting the correct information from a list,

3. or interpreting a diagram to identify or name any of the following features:

   a. Contours of any surface or margin of any surface.

   b. Structural entities such as mamelons, grooves, pits, ridges, fossae, lobes, cingula, etc.

   c. Height of contour and contact areas.

   d. Relative dimensions and shapes.

   e. Any other surface feature.

Furthermore, the student will be able to make comparisons of any of the above features between permanent incisors.

C. Make comparisons among the general characteristics of the permanent incisors, including function, arch position, distinguishing features, etc., by describing them or selecting the correct response from a list, when given the tooth (teeth), or a description of the general characteristic(s).

D. Determine from a diagram or description whether a given permanent incisor is maxillary or mandibular, right or left, or central or lateral.

E. Determine the correct universal number or Palmer notation for a given diagram or description of any permanent incisor.

F. Demonstrate a knowledge of any of the new terms in this unit by defining them, or selecting the correct definition, or application thereof, from a list, when given the term or any of its applications.

G. Demonstrate a knowledge of any of the variations or anomalies in this unit by describing them, or selecting the correct response from a list, when given the particular tooth (teeth), the anomaly, or any of its features or applications.

The student is also responsible for any material which was to have been mastered in previous units.

UNIT # 3
THE PERMANENT INCISORS

I.   **Introduction:**

A.   The permanent incisors are the first and second teeth from the midline, which, along with the canines, comprise the anterior teeth of each quadrant. The incisor closest to the midline is termed the <u>central incisor,</u> while the second tooth from the midline is the <u>lateral incisor.</u> This positions the lateral incisor distal to the central incisor and mesial to the canine.

B.   The central and lateral incisors of the same arch resemble each other more closely than they resemble any incisor of the opposing arch. In size, the maxillary incisor crowns are generally larger than those of the mandibular incisors. In the maxillary arch, the central incisor crown is normally larger than the crown of the lateral incisor. However, in the mandibular arch, the lateral incisor crown and root are generally larger than those of the central incisor, although only very slightly.

C.   The incisors as a group participate in all three of the major functions of the human dentition and have a greater role in esthetics and phonetics than any other group of teeth.

   1.   <u>Mastication</u> - They function by biting, cutting, incising and shearing, thus breaking the food particles into smaller pieces suitable for grinding.

   2.   <u>Esthetics</u> - Not only do the size, shape, color, and manner of placement of incisors directly contribute to a person's appearance, but they provide the support necessary for the normal profile of the lips and face.

   3.   <u>Phonetics</u> - They are necessary for the execution of certain sounds.

D.   Four features which aid in differentiating the crowns of incisors from the crowns of other permanent teeth, include:

   1.   <u>Incisal Edge</u> - This flattened edge, or surface, differs greatly from the single cusp of canines, and the multi-cusped occlusal surfaces of posterior teeth.

   2.   <u>Mamelons</u> - As previously described, mamelons are rounded extensions of enamel on the incisal ridge of recently erupted incisors, and most often are three in number. Mamelons are, however, irregular in number, shape, and prominence. Normally, mamelons wear away soon after the incisors come into active occlusion. However, they are occasionally seen in adult mouths, when the incisors have not been in functional occlusion.

   3.   <u>Position and angulation of marginal ridges</u> - The location and angulation of the marginal ridges of incisors (and canines) contrast markedly with the same features of the marginal ridges of posterior teeth. On incisors, the marginal ridges are the mesial and distal terminations of the lingual surface, and are more or less parallel to the tooth's long axis, while on posterior teeth they are found on the occlusal surface, and are roughly at right angles to the long axis of the tooth.

   4.   <u>Lingual fossa and cingulum</u> - The crowns of the incisors exhibit a concavity which covers roughly the incisal half of the lingual surface. Canines normally have a lingual ridge which creates two fossae on the lingual surface, and posterior teeth display two or more fossae on their occlusal surfaces. The remainder of the lingual surface is occupied by a general convexity which has been previously defined as a cingulum. Canines normally exhibit a cingulum which is more prominent than that of incisors, but posterior teeth have no comparable structure.

II. The Permanent Maxillary Incisors:

A. Introduction:

When compared to the mandibular incisors, those in the maxillary arch have crowns which are generally larger in all dimensions, but especially mesiodistally. The crown area of the maxillary central incisor is normally much greater than that of the maxillary lateral incisor. The lateral incisor crown is similar in form to the crown of the central incisor, only on a smaller size scale in all dimensions.

B. Permanent Maxillary Central Incisor:

    1. General characteristics:

a. Arch position - The maxillary central incisors are the two teeth which are adjacent to the midline in the upper arch. They share a mesial contact area with each other, and have a distal contact with the lateral incisors.

b. Universal number:

Maxillary right central incisor - #8

Maxillary left central incisor - #9

c. General form and function - As viewed from the labial or lingual aspects, the crown is trapezoidal in shape, and the widest mesiodistally of any anterior tooth. As viewed from either proximal aspect, the crown is triangular in shape. The general crown size exceeds that of any other incisor in either arch.

The central incisors' functions in mastication are biting, cutting, incising and shearing. They also play an important role in the esthetics and phonetics functions of the human teeth.

    2. Development Table: (Maxillary central incisor)*

Initiation of calcification .... 3 to 4 months

Completion of enamel .... 4 to 5 years

Eruption .... 7 to 8 years

Completion of root .... 10 years

    3. Labial aspect (of the crown):

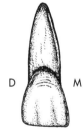

D   M

a. General considerations - The basic geometric shape of the labial surface is trapezoidal, with the longer parallel side at the incisal, and the shorter side at the cervical. Although the crown is longer (incisocervically) than it is wide (mesiodistally), these two dimensions are more nearly equal than for any other permanent incisor. In the maxillary lateral, and even more so in the mandibular incisors, the crown is considerably longer than it is wide.

The labial surface is generally convex in both dimensions, mesiodistally and incisogingivally. The convexity is normally greatest in the cervical third, and tends to more closely approach flatness toward the incisal third.

b. Mesial outline (margin) - The mesial outline of the crown is slightly convex but can be nearly straight, with the crest of curvature at the contact area in the incisal third near the mesioincisal angle. The mesioincisal angle is rather sharp.

*From Wheeler, R.C.: *Dental Anatomy, Physiology and Occlusion* (5th ed.; Philadelphia: W.B. Saunders Company, 1974).

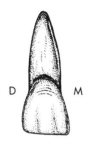

c. Distal outline - This outline is also convex, but more rounded than on the mesial, as is the distoincisal angle. The crest of curvature is associated with the contact area, which is located in the incisal third very near the junction of the incisal and middle thirds, and so is farther cervically than it is on the mesial. Although the cervical half of the mesial and distal outlines is normally convex, either outline can be nearly straight, in comparison to the almost always convex incisal half.

d. Incisal outline - The incisal outline may exhibit mamelons. Without mamelons, the outline is generally straight, and nearly perpendicular to the long axis of the tooth.

e. Cervical margin (or CEJ) - The CEJ curves evenly toward the root. The crown is narrower mesiodistally at the cervical margin than at the incisal.

f. Other considerations:

Developmental depressions - Two straight, shallow depressions, which extend from the incisal edge toward the gingival, and fade out in the middle third. They are termed, mesiolabial and distolabial developmental depressions, and as has already been pointed out, they represent the division of the three labial lobes.

Imbrication lines - Faint, curved lines which roughly parallel the CEJ in the cervical third of the surface. They are not always present.

Height of contour - The height of contour of the labial surface is located in the cervical third.

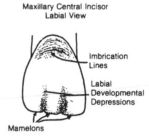

Maxillary Central Incisor
Labial View

4. Lingual aspect:

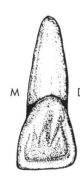

a. General considerations - The lingual surface is also roughly trapezoidal. It is slightly narrower mesiodistally than is the labial, since both mesial and distal surfaces converge slightly toward the lingual, a feature which is also true of all other anterior teeth. It has both convexities and a concavity. The incisal half to two-thirds of the surface is a large, usually shallow, concavity, termed the lingual fossa, while the convex structure in the cervical portion is known as the cingulum.

b. Mesial and distal outlines - These two margins are similar to their labial counterparts, except that they converge slightly more toward the gingival.

c. Incisal margin - The incisal margin is also similar to that of the labial aspect.

d. Cervical margin - The cervical outline has a slightly greater depth of curvature apically than on the labial surface, and is asymmetrical, with its area of maximum curvature offset to the distal.

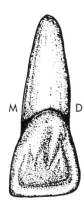

M   D

e. Other considerations:

Lingual fossa - The lingual fossa is the shallow concavity found in the incisal half to two-thirds of the crown, which includes the largest area of the lingual surface. It. is bounded by four convexities; on the mesial and distal by the mesial and distal marginal ridges, on the incisal by the incisal edge, and on the cervical by the cingulum. The fossa is most often smooth. However, there are occasionally rather poorly defined ridges which extend into the cervical portion of the lingual fossa from the cingulum. When present, these ridges may form a "W" shaped pattern.

Cingulum - The cingulum is the bulky convexity located in the cervical portion of the lingual surface. It is generally smooth. Sometimes there is a groove, the linguogingival groove, which separates the cingulum and the lingual fossa. On occasion, there may also be a lingual pit located between the cingulum and fossa. The pit may be found near the center of the linguogingival groove, if that structure is present. The linguogingival groove and lingual pit are much more commonly found on maxillary laterals than on maxillary centrals. However, neither structure is a usual finding on the crown of any permanent incisor.

Marginal ridges - The marginal ridges mark the mesial and distal borders of the lingual fossa, as well as the lingual surface. They are linear, and extend from their respective incisal angles to the cingulum. They are named, by location, mesial and distal marginal ridges.

Height of contour - The lingual crest of curvature is located in the cervical third, at the greatest convexity of the cingulum.

5. Mesial aspect:

a. General considerations - From this aspect, the central incisor crown is roughly triangular in shape, and the incisal edge, at the apex of the triangle, lies over the long axis of the tooth. The mesial surface is generally convex in both dimensions, incisocervically and labiolingually.

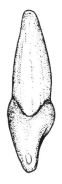

b. Labial outline - The labial outline is convex, with the height of contour and the greatest convexity located in the gingival third. Some specimens may exhibit a flat outline incisal to the crest of curvature.

c. Lingual outline - The lingual margin is somewhat concave in the incisal portion, and convex in the gingival portion, due to the respective contours of the lingual fossa and cingulum. The entire outline may be described as a shallow "S". The crest of curvature of the lingual outline is found in the cervical third at the prominence of the cingulum.

d. Cervical margin - The CEJ curves evenly toward the incisal. It exhibits the greatest depth of curvature of any tooth surface in the mouth.

e. Incisal outline - It is usually pointed, or slightly rounded, in newly erupted incisors, due to the convergence of the labial and lingual surfaces. In teeth with incisal wear, the outline is straight, but slopes from labial to lingual.

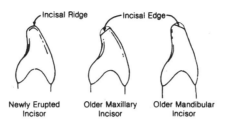

Newly Erupted Incisor   Older Maxillary Incisor   Older Mandibular Incisor

Before proceeding, the difference between two similar terms should be clarified. The incisal ridge is the projection of enamel on newly erupted teeth, which is the incisal termination of the tooth. In a proximal view, it is normally pointed, or slightly rounded. After the tooth enters into occlusion, this ridge is blunted and flattened, resulting in a sloping, straight outline from the proximal aspect. This flattened area is termed the incisal edge.

f. Other considerations:

Height of contour - The mesial height of contour is located in the incisal third at the contact area.

Contact area - The mesial contact area is located in the incisal third, near the incisal margin, and is centered labiolingually. It is roughly ovoid, long incisogingivally, and narrow labiolingually. It is the only proximal area in the maxillary arch where mesial surface contacts mesial surface.

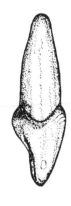

6. Distal aspect:

The distal surface closely resembles the mesial surface, with the following exceptions:

a. The distal surface is generally smaller than the mesial surface, because the incisocervical dimension is shorter.

b. The distal surface is more convex incisogingivally.

c. The cervical margin does not curve as far incisally.

d. Because it contacts the lateral incisor, which is a smaller tooth, the distal contact area is accordingly smaller in size. Its shape is still ovoid, but it is more nearly round than on the mesial. It is also located farther gingivally, still in the incisal third, but very near the junction of the incisal and middle thirds.

7. Incisal aspect:

a. From the incisal aspect, the central incisor's outline is roughly triangular. The incisal edge is relatively straight mesiodistally, and is roughly centered over the root. From this aspect, it can be seen that the lingual surface is narrower mesiodistally than the labial surface. It is also apparent that this tooth and its incisal edge are the widest mesiodistally of any of the permanent incisors.

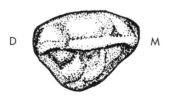

D   M

b. The labial and lingual outlines are convex to differing extents. The labial outline is only slightly convex, while the lingual outline is quite convex, due to the prominence of the cingulum. The labial line angles are more distinct than the lingual line angles. Portions of the lingual fossa and cingulum are visible. Most often, the greatest contour of the cingulum is offset to the distal.

8. Root:

a. The root is single, conical, relatively straight, and tapers to a rounded apex.

b. A horizontal cross section of the root near the cervical line shows a rounded triangular outline. Normally, the root is wider at the labial, which is the base of the triangle, and narrower at the lingual which is the apex. A mid root cross section usually reveals a somewhat ovoid outline, which is wider labiolingually than mesiodistally.

c. The root length is approximately one and a half times the crown length.

9. Variations and Anomalies:

a. Of all the crown surfaces, the lingual exhibits the greatest variation. As previously mentioned, a pit may occasionally be present, and the depth of the fossa has a considerable range.

b. When viewed from the labial or lingual aspects, a wide variation occurs in the amount of convergence of the mesial and distal surfaces toward the cervical. When there is little convergence, the outline of the surface resembles a rectangle, but when great convergence is present, it is more nearly triangular.

c. Root length may vary considerably, but deflections of the root are relatively rare. When the root is exceptionally short, in conjunction with an abnormal contour of the crown, this anomalous condition is referred to as dwarfed root, and the lack of root support may endanger the tooth's longevity in the mouth.

d. Hutchinson's incisors - Congenital syphilis sometimes manifests itself in the central incisor by producing a screwdriver shaped crown, when it is viewed from the labial aspect.

e. Talon cusp - A large accessory cusp on the lingual surface of maxillary incisors characterizes this anomaly. Involved teeth often bear a resemblance to a Phillips screwdriver.

f. The alveolar bone between the roots of the two central incisors is occasionally the site of supernumerary teeth, or extra teeth, known as mesiodens. Cysts may also be found in this area.

C. Permanent Maxillary Lateral Incisor:

1. General characteristics:

a. Arch position - The maxillary lateral incisor is the tooth in each maxillary quadrant of the permanent dentition which is second from the midline. Contact is shared with the permanent central incisor on the mesial, while the distal contact is with the deciduous canine until its exfoliation at about age 12, and then with the permanent canine.

b. Universal number:

Maxillary right lateral incisor - #7

Maxillary left lateral incisor - #10

c. General form and function - The lateral incisor supplements the central incisor in function.

It resembles the central incisor in all aspects, but on a smaller scale. In fact, it is smaller in all measurements, except root length, which is roughly the same. Its relative crown dimensions, and hence its shape, differ slightly from the central, however. It is relatively longer incisocervically and narrower mesiodistally. It also is generally a more round tooth than the central incisor.

The upper lateral incisors display greater variation in form than any other permanent tooth, except the third molars.

2. Development Table: (Maxillary lateral incisor)*

Initiation of calcification .... 1 year

Completion of enamel .... 4 to 5 years

Eruption .... 8 to 9 years

Completion of root .... 11 years

3. Labial aspect:

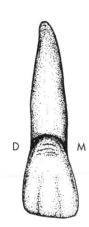

a. Mesial outline - This margin resembles that of the central incisor, but usually is more convex and has a more rounded mesioincisal angle. The crest of curvature, at the contact area, is located farther gingivally in the incisal third, quite near its junction with the middle third.

b. Distal outline - The distal margin is always more rounded than the distal outline of the central incisor, with a more cervically placed crest of curvature, usually at the junction of the incisal and middle thirds. The distoincisal angle is noticeably more rounded than its central incisor counterpart, and also more rounded than its own mesioincisal angle. In fact it is the most rounded incisal angle of any incisor in either arch.

D   M

c. Incisal outline - The incisal outline resembles the central incisor, but it is not so straight, partially because of the greater rounding of the two incisal angles. It exhibits the greatest rounding of any incisor. The number and prominence of mamelons is variable, but two are the most common finding.

d. Cervical outline - The cervical line curves in a regular arc apically, with only slightly less depth than in the central incisor.

e. Other considerations - The labial surface itself is more convex both mesiodistally and incisogingivally than the maxillary central.

Labial developmental depressions and imbrication lines are often present, similar to those of the central incisor.

The labial height of contour is located in the cervical third.

4. Lingual aspect:

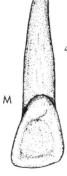

a. Mesial margin - The mesial outline is similar to that of the central incisor.

M   D

b. Distal margin - This margin is also similar to its central incisor counterpart, and the distoincisal angle is much more rounded than is the mesioincisal angle.

c. Incisal outline - The incisal margin is similar to the labial aspect.

d. Cervical outline - The CEJ curves toward the apical, but is offset to the distal.

*From Wheeler, R.C.: *Dental Anatomy, Physiology and Occlusion* (5th ed.; Philadelphia: W.B. Saunders Company, 1974).

e. Other considerations:

The mesial and distal marginal ridges, as well as the cingulum, are relatively more prominent, and the lingual fossa is deeper, when compared to the same structures of the central incisor.

A <u>linguogingival groove</u> is a more common finding in maxillary lateral incisors than in central incisors. A <u>lingual pit</u>, near the center of this groove, is also more common, and when present, is a potential site for caries.

Another groove, which is sometimes found on the lateral, but very rarely on the central incisor, is the <u>linguogingival fissure.</u> This groove usually originates in the lingual pit and extends cervically, and slightly distally, onto the cingulum. It might be helpful to think of the linguogingival fissure as running in a more or less vertical direction, while the linguogingival groove extends in a roughly horizontal direction.

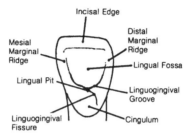

The height of contour is associated with the greatest curvature of the cingulum in the cervical third.

5. Mesial aspect:

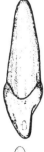

   a. The mesial aspect is very similar to the central incisor, with lessened dimensions.

   b. The contact area is also similar in shape to the contact of the central incisor. It is found in the incisal third very near the junction of the incisal and middle thirds.

   c. The cervical line exhibits less depth of curvature than it does on the mesial of the central incisor.

6. Distal aspect:

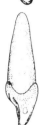

   a. The distal surface is smaller and more convex in all dimensions than the mesial surface.

   b. The contact area is shorter and not as incisally placed, when compared to the mesial contact. It is normally located at the junction of the incisal and middle thirds.

   c. The cervical line shows less curvature incisally than on the mesial surface.

7. Incisal aspect:

   a. From the incisal aspect, the lateral generally resembles the central incisor, except the cingulum is often more prominent.

   b. The lateral incisor also exhibits relatively more convexity labially and lingually than the central incisor, and its outline may approach the rhomboidal appearance of the canine.

8. Root:

a. The lateral incisor root is single, and wider labiolingually than mesiodistally.

b. In comparison to the central, the root is longer in relation to the crown length. In actual length, the root is the same length or slightly shorter than that of the central.

c. The apex is relatively sharper than that of the central, and the apical third may be deflected, and if so it is most often toward the distal.

d. In both cervical and midroot cross sections, the outline is roughly ovoid, wider labiolingually than mesiodistally. The labial dimension is wider mesiodistally than is the lingual.

9. Variations and Anomalies:

a. The incisal portion of the cingulum may exhibit a tubercle.

b. The previously described <u>linguogingival fissure</u> may extend all the way onto the root surface from the adjacent cingulum.

"Peg" Crown

c. Distorted crowns and unusual root curvatures are more commonly seen than with any other incisor.

d. <u>Peg lateral</u> - A diminutive peg-shaped crown form, which is relatively common, and is due to a lack of development of the mesial and distal portions of the crown.

e. Maxillary laterals sometimes are <u>congenitally missing</u>, i.e.: tooth buds do not form (<u>agenesis</u>).

f. The lingual pit of the maxillary lateral may be the entrance site where enamel and dentin have become invaginated in the tooth's pulp cavity, due to a developmental aberrancy called <u>dens in dente</u>.

III. The Permanent Mandibular Incisors:

A. Introduction:

The mandibular incisors are the simplest and least variable teeth in the mouth. They are also the smallest permanent teeth. The central is slightly smaller than the lateral, whereas in the maxillary incisors the central is considerably larger. The mandibular incisors resemble each other to an even greater extent than do the maxillary incisors. Compared to the maxillary incisors, they reveal crowns which are relatively longer incisocervically, and markedly narrower mesiodistally.

B. Permanent Mandibular Central Incisor:

1. General characteristics:

a. Arch position - The mandibular central incisors occupy the position adjacent to the midline in each mandibular quadrant. They share a mesial contact area with each other, while the distal contact is with the permanent lateral incisor.

b. Universal number:

Mandibular right central incisor - #25

Mandibular left central incisor - #24

c. General form and function - The mandibular central incisor normally has the narrowest mesiodistal dimension and the smallest crown size of any permanent tooth. The crown is also quite symmetrical, with mesial and distal halves nearly identical. These teeth function in biting, cutting, incising, and shearing, just as do their maxillary counterparts.

2. Development Table: (Mandibular central incisor)*

Initiation of calcification .... 3 to 4 months

Completion of enamel .... 4 to 5 years

Eruption .... 6 to 7 years

Completion of root .... 9 years

3. Labial aspect:

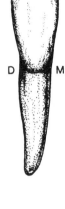

D ● M

a. Mesial outline - The mesial margin normally tapers evenly toward the gingival in a nearly straight line. The mesioincisal angle is quite sharp, normally more so than any of the incisal angles of maxillary incisors. The height of contour is associated with the contact area in the incisal third, very close to the incisal margin.

b. Distal outline - Distally, the outline is straight and almost exactly like the mesial outline, with a similarly sharp distoincisal angle. The height of contour is also in the incisal third.

c. Incisal outline - When present, mamelons most always number three. After incisal wear has obliterated the mamelons, the incisal outline is straight, and at right angles to the long axis of the tooth.

d. Cervical outline - The cervical line is symmetrically curved toward the root.

e. Other considerations - The labial surface is generally convex both mesiodistally and incisogingivally, but not to the extent of the maxillary incisors, especially the maxillary lateral. However, like the maxillary incisors, the convexities are much greater in the cervical third. In fact, in some specimens the labial surface may be quite flat incisal to the height of contour. The surface outline is roughly trapezoidal, which in some cases approaches a rectangular shape.

Developmental depressions and imbrication lines are not normally present. Occasionally, there are very faint depressions which only occur near the incisal margin of the labial surface.

The height of contour is in the cervical third.

4. Lingual aspect:

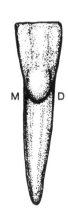

M ● D

a. Mesial, distal and incisal outlines – All three of these margins closely resemble those of the labial aspect.

b. Cervical outline - The CEJ curves evenly toward the root, but is located farther from the incisal edge than it is on the labial surface.

c. Other considerations - The lingual surface is relatively smooth, and its structures are generally less prominent than those of the maxillary incisors. There is usually a slight concavity, or lingual fossa, bordered by indistinct marginal ridges on the mesial and distal. There are normally no grooves, fissures, or pits on the lingual surface.

A cingulum is normally present, although it is not so prominent as in the maxillary incisors.

The height of contour is located in the cervical third of the surface, associated with the greatest convexity of the cingulum.

From Wheeler, R.C.: *Dental Anatomy, Physiology and Occlusion* (5th ed.; Philadelphia: W.B. Saunders Company, 1974).

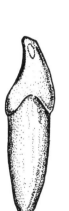

5. Mesial aspect:

    a. Labial outline - The labial margin slopes in a straight to slightly convex line from the incisal ridge to the crest of curvature, and is then convex in the remainder of the gingival third.

    b. Lingual outline - The lingual outline is concave in the incisal two-thirds and convex in the cingulum area, or gingival third.

    c. Incisal outline - The incisal edge is normally straight, but can be slightly rounded, and is located lingual to the center of the root. The profile of the incisal edge has an inclination toward the labial, which is opposite to the lingual slope of the maxillary incisors. This is due to the wear pattern between the upper and lower incisors.

    d. Cervical outline - There is a marked, even curvature incisally of the cervical margin.

    e. Other considerations - The mesial surface is roughly triangular, or wedge shaped, like all other anterior teeth. Unlike the maxillary incisors, the crown appears to be slightly offset toward the lingual.

    The contact area is located about half way from labial to lingual, and in the incisal third, very close to the incisal edge. It has an ovoid shape, which is long incisogingivally and narrow labiolingually.

    The height of contour, at the contact area, is in the incisal third.

6. Distal aspect:

    a. The distal surface is similar in all respects to the mesial, except that the cervical margin curves slightly less toward the incisal. Even the contact area has a similar location, a fact which is unique among incisors.

7. Incisal aspect:

    a. The most notable features from the incisal aspect are the symmetry of the mesial and distal portions, and the straight incisal edge. Unlike the maxillary central, this tooth is roughly four sided, or diamond-shaped, from this aspect, and the tooth is normally wider labiolingually than mesiodistally.

    b. Because the crown is offset toward the lingual, more of the labial surface than the lingual surface is visible from this aspect.

M   D

    c. Even though the central incisor is described as symmetrical from the incisal aspect, careful scrutiny will reveal that the cingulum is very slightly offset toward the distal, an important feature when attempting to distinguish right from left mandibular central incisors.

8. Root:

    a. The root is normally single and straight.

    b. From the labial or lingual aspects, the root is generally symmetrical, and tapers gradually to a relatively sharp apex.

M   D

    c. From the mesial or distal aspects, the root is much wider, and it is slightly convex cervicoapically on both labial and lingual margins. The central portion of the mesial and distal surfaces is usually flattened, or concave. When concave, the surface is said to have a <u>root concavity</u> which is also known as a <u>longitudinal groove</u>. Root concavities are found on the roots of other teeth, and usually extend the majority of the root length, but vary in both length and depth.

d. In cross section at the neck, the outline is roughly a rectangle with rounded corners, but it is slightly wider at the labial than at the lingual. When there are root concavities present, they are reflected as concavities in the mesial and distal outlines. The midroot cross section is similar to the cervical section, only more ovoid.

9. Variations and Anomalies:

a. There is great variability in the lingual inclination of the labial surface of mandibular central incisor specimens.

b. Anomalies are very rare. Occasionally a <u>bifurcated</u> root is found, which means there are two branches, which in mandibular incisors, have labial and lingual locations.

C. Permanent Mandibular Lateral Incisor:

1. General characteristics:

a. Arch position - The mandibular lateral incisor is the second tooth from the midline in each lower quadrant, and it shares a mesial contact area with the central incisor. The distal contact is with the deciduous mandibular canine until that tooth's exfoliation and then contact is shared with the permanent canine.

b. Universal number:

Mandibular right lateral incisor - #26

Mandibular left lateral incisor - #23

c. General form and function - The mandibular lateral incisor is slightly larger in all respects than the mandibular central incisor, but otherwise parallels it very closely in form. It also complements the central in function.

2. Development Table: (Mandibular lateral incisor)*

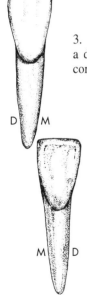

Initiation of calcification .... 3 to 4 months

Completion of enamel .... 4 to 5 years

Eruption .... 7 to 8 years

Completion of root .... 10 years

3. The mandibular lateral incisor so closely resembles the central incisor that a detailed description is unnecessary. Consequently, only the following comparisons need to be made.

a. Labial aspect - The incisal margin may slope slightly gingivally toward the distal, which results in a distoincisal angle that is more rounded than the same angle of the central incisor. This feature creates a slightly shorter distal margin, when compared to the mesial outline. The contact area on the distal is more cervically located than on the mesial, thus creating a more cervically located height of contour on the distal outline. Both heights of contour are still in the incisal third, however.

b. Lingual aspect - The lingual outlines are similar to those of the labial aspect. The structures of the lingual surface are similar to their counterparts on the central incisor, except the cingulum is more offset to the distal, and as a result, the curvature of the cervical line is also offset distally.

D M

M D

From Wheeler, R.C.: *Dental Anatomy, Physiology and Occlusion* (5th ed.; Philadelphia: W.B. Saunders Company, 1974).

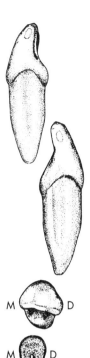

c. Mesial and distal aspects - These two surfaces are similar to their counterparts on the central incisor, with a few minor exceptions. The lateral's distal surface is slightly shorter incisocervically than the mesial surface. Both cervical line curvatures are slightly less than their counterparts in the central, and as would be expected, the mesial cervical line shows greater incisal curvature than does the distal. The distal contact area, and hence the height of contour, is more cervically located than on the mesial. Although still in the incisal third, the distal contact area is very near the junction of the incisal and middle thirds, and is the most cervically located of any mandibular incisor contact.

d. Incisal aspect - From this view, the incisal edge is not straight mesiodistally, as it is in the central; rather it curves toward the lingual in its distal portion. Furthermore, the lingual contour (cingulum) appears displaced toward the distal. These factors give the crown the appearance of being slightly twisted on its root. These are the best identifying features, when differentiating this tooth from the central incisor.

e. Root - Root length is normally a little greater than in the central incisor. The root is also slightly thicker and wider. Root concavities may be found on the mesial and distal root surfaces, and if present, the concavity in the distal is usually more pronounced.

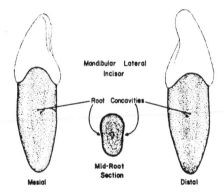

4. Variations and Anomalies:

   a. Anomalies are rare, but occasionally a bifurcated root is found.

Maxillary Right Central Incisor

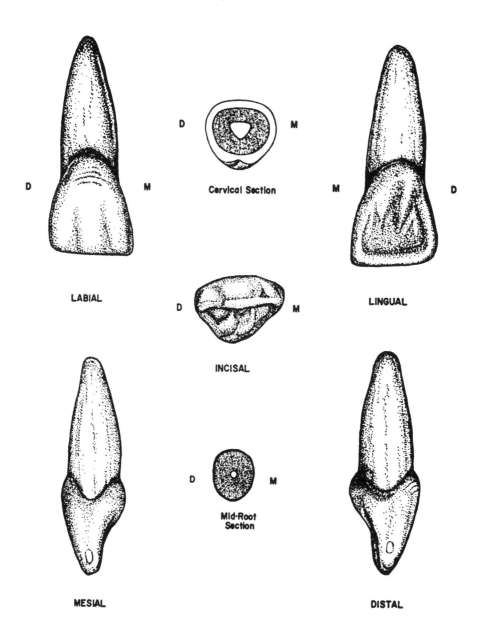

D   M   Cervical Section

LABIAL

D   M   INCISAL

LINGUAL

D   M   Mid-Root Section

MESIAL

DISTAL

Maxillary Right Lateral Incisor

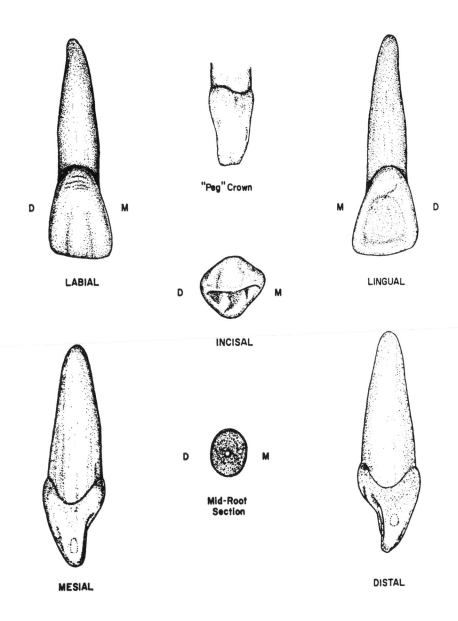

D   M

LABIAL

"Peg" Crown

D   M

INCISAL

M   D

LINGUAL

D   M

**Mid-Root
Section**

MESIAL

DISTAL

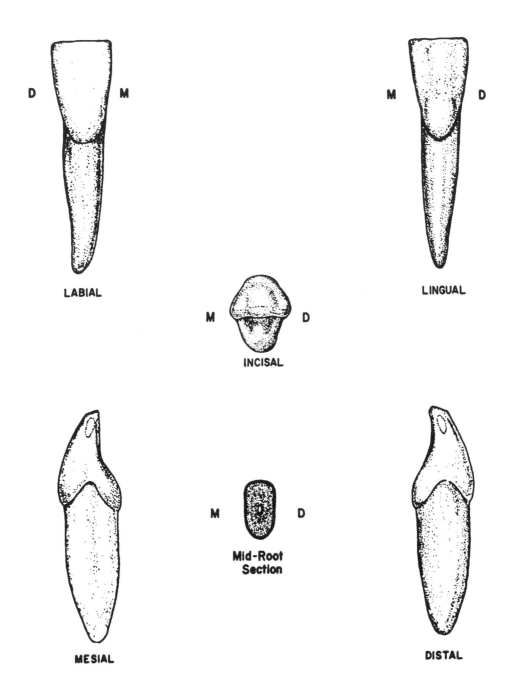

LABIAL

LINGUAL

M   D

INCISAL

M   D

Mid-Root
Section

MESIAL

DISTAL

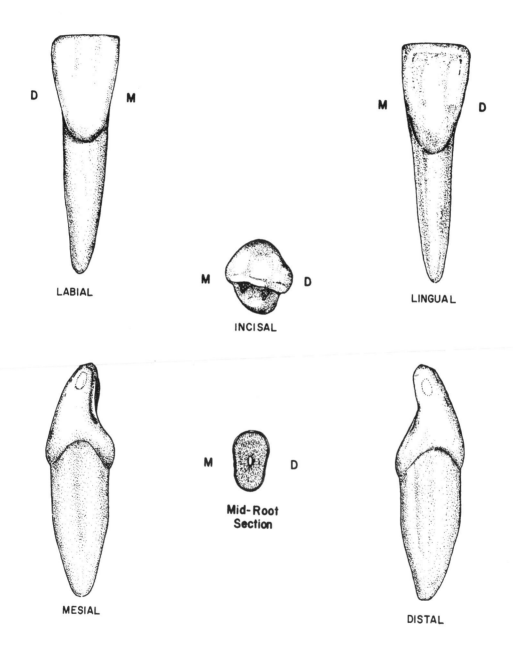

LABIAL

INCISAL

LINGUAL

MESIAL

Mid-Root
Section

DISTAL

UNIT # 4

I. **Reading Assignment:**

Unit # 4 (The Permanent Canines)

II. **Specific Objectives:**

At the completion of this unit, the student will be able to:

A.   List the appropriate age(s) concerning developmental chronology of the permanent canines found in the development tables, or select the appropriate age(s) from a list, when given a certain developmental feature. The student should also be able to compare these ages between the canines.

B.   Demonstrate a knowledge of the morphology of each surface of the crown, as well as the root, of each permanent canine by:

    1.   describing,

    2.   selecting the correct information from a list,

    3.   or interpreting a diagram to identify or name any of the following features:

        a. Contours of any surface or margin of any surface.

        b. Structural entities such as grooves, pits, ridges, fossae, lobes, cingula, etc.

        c. Height of contour and contact areas.

        d. Relative dimensions and shape.

        e. Any other surface feature.

Furthermore, the student will be able to make comparisons of any of these features between the canines.

C.   Make comparisons between permanent incisors and canines, where appropriate, by selecting the correct response from a list.

D.   Make comparisons between the general characteristics of the permanent canines, including function, arch position, distinguishing features, etc., by describing them, or selecting the correct response from a list, when given the tooth (teeth), or a description of the general characteristic(s).

E.   Determine from a diagram or description whether a given permanent canine is maxillary or mandibular, or right or left.

F.   Determine the correct universal number or Palmer notation for a given diagram or description of any permanent canine.

G.   Demonstrate a knowledge of any of the new terms in this unit by defining them, or selecting the correct definition, or application thereof, from a list, when given the term, or any of its applications.

H.   Demonstrate a knowledge of any of the variations or anomalies in this unit by describing them, or selecting the correct response from a list, when given the particular tooth (teeth), the anomaly, or any of its features or applications.

The student is also responsible for any material which was to have been mastered in previous units.

THE PERMANENT CANINES

I. **The Permanent Canines**

   A. Introduction:

      1. The canines are the most important teeth in the mouth of carnivores, and are the "fangs" of many animals. In fact, the name, canine, is derived from the Latin term for dog.

      2. The human permanent canines (or cuspids) in each arch have a similar appearance and function. They are often called the "cornerstones of the mouth", since they are intermediary between the incisors and posterior teeth in function, form, and arch position.

         a. In <u>function</u>, the canine's role in mastication is mainly tearing, which is intermediate between the incising of the other anterior teeth, and the grinding of the posterior teeth. They also contribute greatly to the cosmetic and facial support function, and play a part in phonetics as well.

         b. In <u>form,</u> they have the same general wedge shape as the incisors, when viewed from a proximal aspect. However, when viewed from the facial, they look like premolars. They exhibit biting edges, cingula, and marginal ridges which are similar to those of incisors, while the facial ridge and cusp are features common to posterior teeth.

         c. In <u>arch position</u>, they are the third tooth from the midline in each quadrant, and are positioned as a cornerstone between the more or less laterally positioned incisors and the anteroposteriorly positioned premolars and molars. This location is important to an individual's appearance, since the canines play a major role in the support of the facial muscles.

      3. The canines exhibit the greatest combined crown plus root length in each arch, and their root is very firmly anchored in alveolar bone. The thick facial plate of bone overlying the canine root is termed the <u>canine eminence</u>. Because of this bony support, and the length of the root, the canines are usually the most steadfast teeth in the mouth.

   B. Permanent Maxillary Canine:

      1. General characteristics:

         a. Arch position - The permanent maxillary canine replaces the deciduous maxillary canine, and is located third from the midline in each maxillary quadrant. The canine shares a mesial contact with the maxillary lateral incisor, and contacts the maxillary first premolar on the distal.

         b. Universal number:

            Maxillary right canine - #6

            Maxillary left canine - #11

         c. General form and function - As already pointed out, the canine's function in mastication is mainly tearing and piercing and they also function in esthetics and speech. The general crown form is pentagonal when viewed from the labial or lingual aspect, and triangular when viewed from the proximals. The crown exhibits one rather sharp cusp incisally which has two biting edges, in comparison to the single and relatively straight incisal edge of the incisors. The crown is bulky in comparison to the incisors, especially labiolingually, which gives it the appearance of strength.

2. Comparisons to the maxillary central incisor:

a. Incisogingivally, the crown length is about the same, or even slightly shorter, than that of the central incisor.

b. Mesiodistally, the canine crown is noticeably narrower.

c. Labiolingually, the crown is considerably wider than that of the central incisor.

d. The root is longer, and the combined crown plus root length is greater in the canine.

e. The cingulum shows greater development, and it is a much stronger tooth than the central incisor.

f. The middle labial lobe of the canine is much better developed, which is partially responsible for the greater convexity of the canine's facial surface.

3. Development Table (Maxillary canine)*

Initiation of calcification .... 4 to 5 months

Completion of enamel .... 6 to 7 years

Eruption .... 11 to 12 years

Completion of root .... 13 to 15 years

4. Labial aspect:

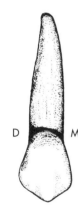

D   M

a. General considerations - The labial surface is convex in all directions, but the curvature is more pronounced mesiodistally. The general outline of the surface is pentagonal.

b. Mesial outline - The mesial margin is usually convex from the mesial contact area to the cervical line, with a rounded mesioincisal angle. The height of contour of this margin is at the contact area, which is located at the junction of the incisal and middle thirds.

c. Distal margin - The distal margin is shorter than the mesial margin, and is usually concave between the distal contact area and the cervical line. It also has a more rounded incisal angle. The height of contour, at the contact area, is in the middle third.

d. Incisal margin - The incisal margin is divided into two components by the tip of the cusp, and they are termed the mesioincisal and distoincisal slopes (or mesial and distal cusp ridges). Prior to attrition, the mesioincisal slope is normally the shorter of the two, and also slopes to a lesser degree. Nevertheless, the tip of the cusp is located in line with the center of the root.

With normal attritional wear, the cusp tip moves to the distal, thus lengthening the mesioincisal slope and shortening the distoincisal slope.

Usually the cusp tip also extends past the plane of occlusion of the other teeth in the arch. This extension may be as much as a millimeter or two, and reflects the evolution of the human canine from the carnivorous animal fang.

e. Cervical outline - The CEJ is quite evenly curved toward the root.

f. Other considerations - A labial ridge transcends the middle of the surface in an incisocervical direction, and is most prominent in the incisal portion. This ridge represents a greater development of the middle labial

*From Wheeler, R.C.: Dental Anatomy, Physiology and Occlusion (5th ed.; Philadelphia: W.B. Saunders Company, 1974).

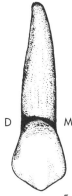

lobe, as compared to the mesial and distal labial lobes. It is responsible for the greater mesiodistal convexity of the incisal two-thirds of the labial surface, when compared to the incisors.

Separating the three lobes and lying on either side of the labial ridge in the incisal portion of the labial surface are two faint concavities, termed mesiolabial and distolabial developmental depressions. In newly erupted canines, these depressions may extend onto the two incisal slopes, thus creating a slightly concave, or notched area, when viewed from the facial.

Imbrication lines can often be found in the cervical third of the surface, especially in newly erupted teeth, but mamelons are ordinarily not present on the incisal outline

The height of contour is located in the cervical third of the surface.

5. Lingual aspect:

a. Mesial, distal, and incisal outlines - These margins are similar to those of the labial aspect.

b. Cervical outline - The cervical line curves asymmetrically toward the apex with a slight offset to the distal.

c. Other considerations - The mesiodistal dimension of the lingual surface is less than that of the labial surface, since the mesial and distal surfaces converge slightly toward the lingual.

The cingulum is bulky, and normally smooth. It shows greater development than the cingulum of the maxillary central incisor. The marginal ridges are also prominent.

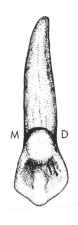

The incisal half of the surface is relatively smooth, but does exhibit faint landmarks. There is normally a lingual ridge extending incisogingivally in the center of this area, with shallow mesiolingual and distolingual fossae between it and the prominent marginal ridges.

The cingulum and incisal half of the lingual surface are on rare occasions separated by a linguogingival groove, which in some cases may contain a lingual pit near its center. When present, the groove is normally quite shallow. The lingual pit may be present, even when the groove is absent. Nevertheless, the presence of a groove or pit is not very common.

The lingual height of contour is associated with the greatest convexity of the cingulum in the cervical third.

6. Mesial aspect:

a. General considerations - The mesial surface is convex in all dimensions, and is wider labiolingually than the mesial surface of any of the incisors. Like other anterior teeth, it is triangular in shape.

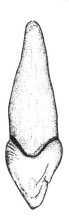

b. Labial outline - The labial margin is convex incisocervically, with the crest of curvature in the cervical third. This convexity is slightly greater than for the same outline of the maxillary incisors.

c. Lingual outline - The lingual outline is concave in the incisal half, and convex in the cingulum area, or gingival half, but less so than on incisor crowns because of the lingual ridge. The height of contour is in the cervical third.

d. Cervical outline - The cervical line is curved evenly toward the incisal, with the greatest extent of curvature directly beneath the incisal edge.

e. Incisal outline - The incisal edge is thick, and from this aspect, has an outline which slopes from labial to lingual, like the maxillary incisors.

f. Other considerations - The contact area is located at the junction of the middle and incisal thirds, about midway between the labial and lingual surfaces. It has an ovoid shape, which is longer incisogingivally than labiolingually.

The height of contour of the mesial surface is located at the contact area, at the junction of the incisal and middle thirds.

7. Distal aspect: The distal surface is similar to the mesial surface, with the following exceptions:

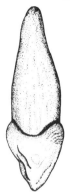

a. The distal surface is generally smaller, with resultant shorter labial and lingual margins.

b. The cervical margin exhibits less curvature incisally than it does on the mesial surface.

c. The lingual outline of the distal marginal ridge is likely to be more ir-regular than the outline of the mesial marginal ridge.

d. The contact area is more circular than on the mesial, and is located at a more cervical level which is in the middle third. Although a different shape, it occupies about the same sized area as does the mesial contact.

e. A concavity is usually present in the cervical half of the distal surface.

f. The height of contour is located at a more cervical level, and is associ-ated with the contact area in the middle third.

8. Incisal aspect:

a. From the incisal, the maxillary canine is generally convex in both its labial and lingual outlines. The tooth's strength is exhibited by the thicker labiolingual dimension, when compared to the maxillary incisors.

b. From this aspect, the canine crown has an asymmetrical diamond shaped outline. The mesial half is thicker labiolingually and more convex, while the distal portion is thinner and exhibits a slight concavity in its labial and/or lingual outline. The cingulum is offset to the distal from this view.

c. The greater development of the middle labial lobe is also evident from the incisal aspect, and contributes to the increased convexity of the labial outline, when compared to the maxillary incisors.

9. Root:

a. The root is single, and normally the longest root of any tooth in the mouth.

b. From all aspects, the root tapers gradually to a sharp, or slightly blunted apex.

c. The root is generally wider labiolingually than mesiodistally. Both lin-gual and labial surfaces are convex, while the mesial and distal surfaces are convex or slightly flattened. The root, like the crown, exhibits mesial and distal surfaces which converge toward the lingual. Thus, the labial root surface is wider mesiodistally than the lingual root surface.

d. In cross section at the neck, the root is roughly ovoid, with convex labial and lingual outlines, but with mesial and distal outlines which are flattened or only slightly convex. Furthermore, the outline is wider mesiodistally at the labial than at the lingual. The mid root section is similar, except that the mesial and distal outlines are most likely to be convex.

10. Variations and Anomalies:

   a. Crown form does not vary widely, although the sharpness of the cusp tip has considerable range.

   b. On rare occasions, the lingual surface may exhibit a tubercle which is located near the most incisal level of the cingulum. When a tubercle is present, a lingual pit is often associated with it.

   c. Root form is subject to variations. There may be several curvatures along its length. If curved in the apical third, the deflection is most commonly to the distal.

   d. Since the maxillary canine normally erupts after the maxillary premolars, its space is sometimes partially closed. It may then erupt well to the labial or lingual of the other teeth, or not erupt at all, in which case it is considered to be <u>impacted</u>.

C. Permanent Mandibular Canine:

   1. General characteristics:

      a. Arch position - The mandibular canine is the third tooth from the midline in each lower quadrant, and is the replacement for the deciduous mandibular canine. The mesial contact is shared with the mandibular lateral incisor, while distally it contacts the mandibular first premolar.

      b. Universal Number:

      Mandibular right canine - #27

      Mandibular left canine - #22

      c. General form and function - Form and function are similar to those of the maxillary canine.

   2. Comparisons with the maxillary canine:

      a. The crown is as long, or longer incisocervically, when compared to the maxillary canine.

      b. The mesiodistal and labiolingual dimensions of both crown and root are normally less in the mandibular canine.

      c. The root is usually shorter than the maxillary canine's, but in some cases, may be as long. The total crown plus root length is approximately the same for the two canines.

      d. The lingual surface and its structures are less well developed than in the maxillary canine. In fact, the form of the lingual surface is more closely allied to that of the mandibular incisors, even with the presence of a lingual ridge.

      e. The cusp of the mandibular canine is not so well developed, nor is its tip normally as sharp mesiodistally as in the maxillary canine.

      f. The labial surface is generally not so convex as in the maxillary canine. This is especially true in the incisal two-thirds of the surface. However, it may be more convex mesiodistally in the cervical third.

   3. Development Table: (Mandibular canine)*

   Initiation of calcification .... 4 to 5 months

   Completion of enamel .... 6 to 7 years

   Eruption .... 9 to 10 years

   Completion of root .... 12 to 14 years

---

*From Wheeler, R.C.: *Dental Anatomy, Physiology and Occlusion* (5th ed.; Philadelphia: W.B. Saunders Company, 1974).

63

4. Labial aspect:

a. General considerations - Even though the dimensions differ, the general outline of the tooth from the labial aspect is pentagonal, like the maxillary canine. As pointed out, the labial surface is generally not so convex (except mesiodistally in the cervical third) as the maxillary canine, but is generally more convex than in the mandibular incisors.

b. Mesial outline - The mesial outline is pretty much a straight line from the mesial contact to the cervical line, with an obtuse mesioincisal angle. The crest of curvature of this margin is near the mesioincisal angle, and is associated with the contact area in the incisal third.

c. Distal outline - Distally, the outline is convex incisocervically, with a more rounded distoincisal angle. The distal margin is shorter than the mesial margin. The height of contour, which is associated with the contact area at the junction of the incisal and middle thirds, is more cervically located than on the mesial outline.

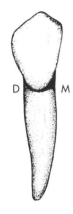

d. Incisal outline - The cusp is not as long or the tip as sharp as the maxillary canine cusp. The distoincisal slope is normally longer, and its angulation cervically is much steeper than the mesioincisal slope exhibits.

Since the distoincisal slope of the mandibular canine normally occludes with the mesioincisal slope of the maxillary canine, the wear pattern is reflected in a mesial displacement of the cusp tip of the mandibular canine, and a lengthening of its distoincisal slope. However, prior to attrition, the cusp tip is located directly over the root center, as in the maxillary canine.

e. Cervical outline - The cervical line is evenly curved toward the root.

f. Other considerations - The labial surface appears to be much longer incisocervically than the maxillary canine, and in fact, it is as long, or slightly longer. However, the main reasons for this appearance are its narrower mesiodistal dimension, and the more incisal location of the contact areas.

The labial ridge is not as prominent as in the maxillary canine. Developmental depressions are positioned and named like those of the incisors and maxillary canine, but imbrication lines are normally absent.

The labial height of contour is located in the cervical third.

5. Lingual aspect:

a. Mesial, distal, and incisal outlines - These margins mimic those of the labial aspect.

b. Cervical margin - The cervical line exhibits a greater depth of curvature than on the labial, and it is uneven, with the greatest curvature offset to the distal.

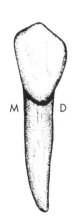

c. Other considerations - The lingual surface is generally smoother and lacking in anatomic detail, when compared to the maxillary canine. The cingulum does not extend so far incisally, and it and the marginal ridges are not so prominent. There is normally a less pronounced lingual ridge, and shallow distolingual and mesiolingual fossae usually occur in the incisal portion of the surface. There are rarely any grooves, pits, or tubercles on the lingual surface.

As is the case with other anterior teeth, the lingual surface is slightly narrower mesiodistally than the labial surface.

The lingual height of contour is associated with the greatest prominence of the cingulum in the cervical third.

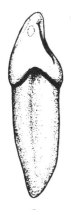

6. Mesial aspect:

a. Labial margin - The entire labial outline is convex, with the greatest rounding at the height of contour in the cervical third.

b. Lingual margin - The lingual outline is similar to that of the maxillary canine, except the cingulum convexity is less prominent and located farther cervically.

c. Incisal margin - The outline of the incisal ridge is thinner labiolingually.

d. Cervical margin - The CEJ is quite evenly curved incisally.

e. Other considerations - The mesial surface is roughly triangular in shape like the maxillary canine, but noticeably narrower labiolingually. The surface contour is basically convex labiolingually, but incisocervically there is usually a flattening between the cervical line and the contact area.

The contact area is located in the incisal third, about midway between the labial and lingual surfaces. It is ovoid, and wider incisogingivally than labiolingually.

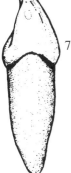

7. Distal aspect:

a. The distal is similar to the mesial surface in all respects, except that it is slightly smaller in all dimensions.

b. The contact area, and thus the height of contour, are found at a more cervical level at the junction of the incisal and middle thirds. It also has a different outline which approaches a circular shape.

c. There is no incisocervical flattening on the distal surface, as there is on the mesial surface.

8. Incisal aspect:

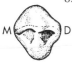

a. Although the relative dimensions differ, this tooth is similar to the maxillary canine, when viewed from the incisal. The crown is thicker labiolingually toward the mesial, and the cingulum is offset to the distal. The labial outline is more convex mesiodistally than in the mandibular incisors.

9. Root:

a. The root is normally single, fairly straight, and the longest root in the mandibular arch.

b. Like most other anterior teeth, it is narrower mesiodistally than labiolingually. The lingual portion is narrower mesiodistally than is the labial. Both labial and lingual surfaces are convex, while the mesial and distal surfaces are flattened or concave. When concavities are present, they extend cervicoapically along the root, and in some cases run the entire root length. As in the mandibular incisors, they are named <u>root concavities</u>, or <u>longitudinal grooves.</u>

c. In cross section at the neck, the outline is roughly a flattened ovoid, wider labiolingually, and wider mesiodistally at the labial than the lingual. If root concavities are present, the proximal outline will be concave. The mid root section is similar, but the mesial and distal surfaces are more likely to be flattened rather than concave.

10. Variations and Anomalies:

a. Crown form is not greatly variable.

b. Irregularly curved roots are occasionally seen, and <u>bifurcated</u> roots, with labial and lingual branches, are also possible.

Maxillary Right Canine

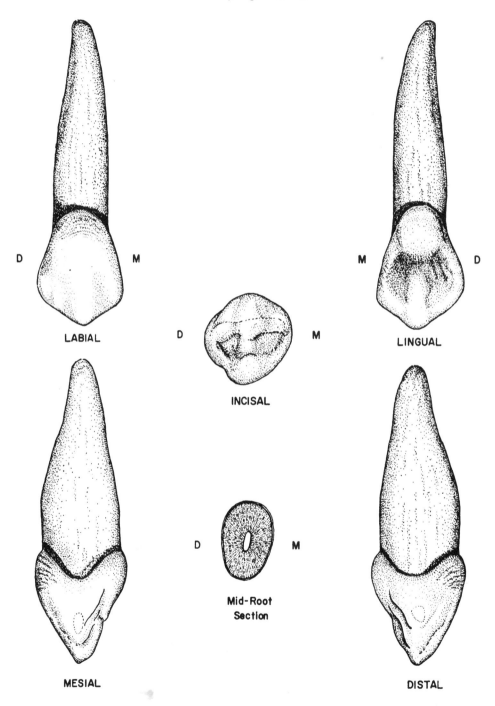

D   M

LABIAL

D   M

INCISAL

M   D

LINGUAL

MESIAL

D   M

Mid-Root
Section

DISTAL

Mandibular Right Canine

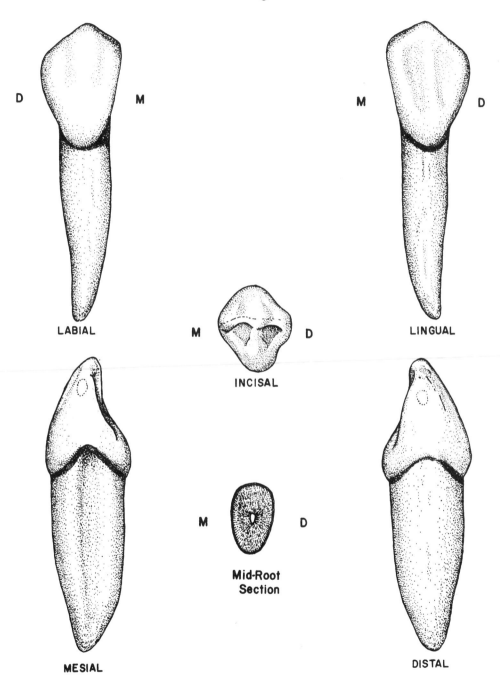

D   M

LABIAL

M   D

LINGUAL

M   D

INCISAL

M   D

Mid-Root Section

MESIAL

DISTAL

Comparison of Incisal Slopes
In Newly Erupted and Worn Canines

**Maxillary Right Canine
Newly Erupted**

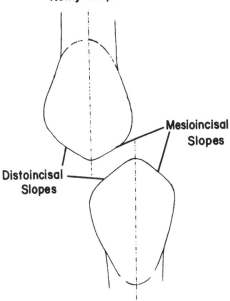

**Mesioincisal
Slopes**

**Distoincisal
Slopes**

**Mandibular Right Canine
Newly Erupted**

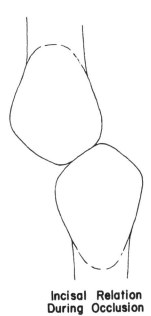

**Incisal Relation
During Occlusion**

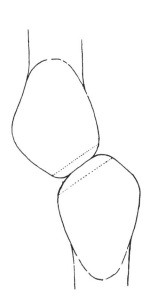

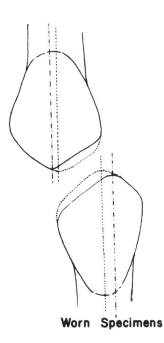

Worn Specimens

UNIT # 5

I.   **Reading Assignment:**

Unit # 5 (The Permanent Maxillary Premolars)

II.   **Specific Objectives:**

At the completion of this unit, the student will be able to:

A.   List the appropriate age(s) concerning the developmental chronology of the maxillary premolars found in the development tables, or select the appropriate age(s) from a list, when given a certain developmental feature. The student should also be able to compare these facts between the maxillary premolars.

B.   Demonstrate a knowledge of the morphology of each surface of the crown, as well as the root, of each permanent maxillary premolar by:

    1.   describing,

    2.   selecting the correct information from a list,

    3.   or interpreting a diagram to identify or name any of the following features:

      a. Contours of any surface, or margin of any surface.

      b. Structural entities such as grooves, pits, ridges, inclined planes, cusps, fossae, lobes, etc.

      c. Height of contour and contact areas.

      d. Relative dimensions and shape.

      e. Any other surface feature.

Furthermore, the student will be able to make comparisons of any of these features between the maxillary premolars.

C.   Make comparisons between maxillary premolars and other permanent teeth, where appropriate, by selecting the correct response from a list.

D.   Make comparisons between the general characteristics of the maxillary premolars, including function, arch position, distinguishing features, etc., by describing them, or selecting the correct response from a list, when given the tooth (teeth), or a description of the general characteristic(s).

E.   Determine from a diagram or description whether a given maxillary premolar is first or second, or right or left.

F.   Determine the correct universal number or Palmer notation for a given diagram or description of any maxillary premolar.

G.   Demonstrate a knowledge of any of the new terms in this unit by defining them, or selecting the correct definition, or application thereof, from a list, when given the term, or any of its applications.

H.   Demonstrate a knowledge of any of the variations or anomalies in this unit by describing them, or selecting the correct response from a list, when given the particular tooth (teeth), the anomaly, or any of its features or applications.

The student is also responsible for any material which was to have been mastered in previous units.

UNIT # 5
PERMANENT MAXILLARY PREMOLARS

I. **Permanent Premolars:**

A. Introduction:

1. Eight premolars are found in the permanent dentition, with four per arch and two in each quadrant. They are located in the fourth and fifth positions from the midline, which places them between the canines and molars. The premolars are designated as <u>first premolar</u> or <u>second premolar</u>, by noting their position relative to the midline, with the first premolar closest.

2. Along with the molars, the premolars comprise the group of teeth collectively referred to as posterior teeth. As previously indicated, major anatomical and functional differences exist between the posterior teeth and the anterior teeth.

3. The term "bicuspid" is often used when referring to premolars. This term, which signifies "two cusps", is a somewhat inaccurate description for the group as a whole, as further study of the premolars will reveal.

4. Just as the canine is intermediate between the posterior teeth and the other anterior teeth, the premolars are transitional between the canine and the molars in function, form, and arch position.

a. In <u>function</u>, the premolars mainly supplement the grinding of the molars during mastication, but there is still a tearing and piercing component, similar to that of the canine. The premolars contribute less to esthetics and phonetics than do the anterior teeth, but provide a greater share of these functions than do molars.

b. In <u>form,</u> the major structural changes from the canine include the increased number of cusps, marginal ridge location, root structure, and presence of an occlusal surface. The premolars always exhibit one facial cusp like the canines, but the number of lingual cusps can range from none to two. Most commonly there is one lingual cusp, hence the derivation of the term bicuspid.

c. In <u>arch position</u>, the premolars occupy the fourth and fifth positions from the midline, thus leaving three anterior teeth mesial, and three molars distal to them in each quadrant.

5. The two maxillary premolars are much more alike in size, shape, and function than are the mandibular premolars.

6. Because premolars erupt in the position previously occupied by the deciduous molars, they are succedaneous teeth. They are the only succedaneous teeth which have a name different than that of the deciduous teeth they replace.

II. **The Permanent Maxillary Premolars:**

A. Introduction:

Maxillary premolars possess a number of general characteristics which aid in differentiating them from other posterior teeth, especially from the premolars in the mandibular arch.

1. Maxillary first and second premolars are much more similar to each other than are the mandibular premolars.

2. In the maxillary arch, the first premolar is generally a little larger than the second premolar, while in the mandible the first premolar is considerably smaller.

70

3.   The crowns of maxillary premolars are normally wider buccolingually than mesiodistally, while the mandibular premolars' buccolingual and mesiodistal crown dimensions are approximately equal.

4.   Maxillary premolars possess two cusps of nearly equal size. The mandibular premolars may have more than two cusps, and the lingual cusps are normally less prominent than the facial cusps.

5.   When viewed from either proximal surface, the crown profile of the maxillary premolars shows virtually no lingual inclination, and thus is pretty much centered over the root. In contrast, the crowns of the mandibular premolars are heavily inclined and offset toward the lingual.

6.   The maxillary first premolar is the only premolar which normally exhibits two root branches.

B.   The Permanent Maxillary First Premolar:

1.   General characteristics:

a. Arch position - The maxillary first premolar is the fourth permanent tooth from the midline. It has a mesial contact with the permanent maxillary canine, and a distal contact with the second premolar. It replaces the deciduous maxillary first molar, and hence is a succedaneous tooth.

b. Universal number:

Maxillary right first premolar - #5

Maxillary left first premolar - #12

c. General form and function - The outline from the occlusal aspect roughly resembles a hexagonal, or six-sided figure, while the general shape from the proximal aspects is trapezoidal. From the facial aspect, the shape is pentagonal and quite similar to that of a maxillary canine. The first premolar exhibits two very similar cusps, plus two root branches in the majority of specimens.

In mastication, the first premolar functions basically as a grinding tooth, and contributes to the esthetics and phonetics roles as well.

2.   Development Table: (Maxillary first premolar)*

Initiation of calcification .... 1 1/ 2 - 1 3/ 4 yrs.

Completion of enamel .... 5 - 6 yrs.

Eruption .... 10 - 11 yrs.

Completion of root .... 12 - 13 yrs.

3.   Buccal aspect:

a. General considerations - From the facial aspect, the pentagonally shaped crown bears a close resemblance to those of both the maxillary canine and second premolar. However, the canine crown is somewhat larger in size, with a more prominent cusp tip, and the crown of the second premolar is smaller, with a less prominent cusp tip. The occlusocervical dimension of the crown is less than for any anterior tooth, but greater than that of the second premolar or any molar.

b. Mesial margin - The mesial margin joins the mesio-occlusal slope to create an obtuse mesio-occlusal angle. The contour of the mesial outline is shallowly concave from the contact area to the cervical line. The crest of

D   M

*From Wheeler, R.C.: *Dental Anatomy, Physiology and Occlusion* (5th ed.; Philadelphia: W.B. Saunders Company, 1974).

curvature at the contact area is located near the junction of the occlusal and middle thirds.

c. Distal margin - The distal is slightly shorter, but otherwise is much the same as the mesial margin, but the disto-occlusal angle is a little less prominent, and the cervical concavity is not as deep. The crest of curvature is also slightly more cervically located.

d. Occlusal outline - The occlusal margin of this tooth is, similar to the incisal margin of the maxillary canine. The facial cusp tip is pronounced, although it is not as prominent as is the maxillary canine's. The cusp tip divides the occlusal outline into two unequal portions. The mesio-occlusal slope is longer and straighter, while the disto-occlusal slope is shorter and more curved. The cusp tip is thus offset slightly toward the distal. This relationship of the occlusal slopes normally exists prior to attrition, and of course wear may alter it.

Occasionally, the developmental depressions pass over the occlusal margin, with a resultant concavity, or notch in the outline of each of the occlusal slopes.

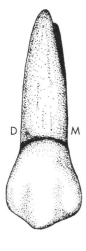

e. Cervical outline - The CEJ is evenly convex toward the apex, but the depth of curvature is generally less than that found in the anterior teeth.

f. Other considerations - The most notable feature on the buccal surface is the buccal ridge. It extends about halfway along the surface from the tip of the buccal cusp toward the cervical line, and is the result of the greater development of the middle buccal lobe. It is comparable to the labial ridge of the canines.

Mesiobuccal and distobuccal developmental depressions are present on each side of the buccal ridge, and appear to divide the occlusal portion of the buccal surface into vertical thirds, corresponding to the three buccal lobes.

In the cervical third of the surface, imbrication lines are also a common finding.

The height of contour is located in the cervical third of the surface.

4. Lingual aspect:

a. General considerations - The lingual surface of the crown is smoothly convex in all directions. There is no clearly defined lingual ridge.

The crown tapers toward the lingual, so the tooth is narrower mesiodistally at the lingual than at the buccal. In fact, the lingual surface is smaller than the buccal surface in all dimensions.

Since the lingual cusp is shorter than the buccal cusp, the tips of both are visible from the lingual aspect. However, the two cusp tips do not fall on the same line, since the lingual cusp tip is noticeably offset to the mesial, which is opposite to the distal placement of the buccal cusp tip.

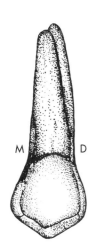

b. Mesial and distal outlines - The proximal outlines are normally somewhat convex, and shorter than the same outlines of the buccal surface. However, the mesial outline may be concave if the mesial concavity is severe.

c. Occlusal outline - The lingual cusp tip is not as sharply pointed as the buccal cusp tip. It is offset toward the mesial, making the mesio-occlusal slope shorter than the disto-occlusal slope. It is shorter than the buccal cusp, usually by as much as one millimeter, or occasionally even more. In fact, it is the shortest of the four maxillary premolar cusps.

d. Cervical outline - The cervical line is curved symmetrically toward the apex.

e. Other considerations - No developmental depressions, grooves, or pits are normally found on this surface.

The lingual height of contour is normally located in the middle third.

5. Mesial aspect:

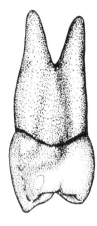

a. General considerations - The general shape of the mesial surface is trapezoidal, with the longer parallel side located at the cervical.

b. Buccal margin - The buccal outline is generally convex, with the height of contour in the cervical third.

c. Lingual margin - Lingually, the outline takes the form of an even arc, with the height of contour in the middle third.

d. Occlusal margin - The occlusal margin is irregularly concave, and the majority of it is made up of the <u>mesial marginal ridge</u>. A prominent <u>mesial marginal groove</u> is usually present indenting the occlusal margin almost two-thirds of the way from the buccal to the lingual outline.

e. Cervical margin - The cervical line is most often irregularly convex toward the occlusal, due to the mesial concavity, but on occasional specimens it has an even convexity. The depth of curvature is less than that found on any anterior tooth except the distal of the canine, where the two are equal.

f. Other considerations - From this aspect, it is easy to observe the difference in height between the two cusp tips.

<u>Mesial concavity</u> - A unique feature of the mesial surface of the maxillary first premolar is the mesial concavity. This depressed area is variable in its extent. Most often, it is limited to the middle portion of the cervical third, but some specimens exhibit an extension which may reach as far as the middle portion of the mesiobuccal line angle area. This landmark is a relatively consistent way to distinguish the maxillary first premolar from the second premolar, which usually lacks it.

The mesial height of contour is associated with the contact area, near the junction of the middle and occlusal thirds. The contact area is roughly circular in shape and is offset to the buccal.

6. Distal aspect:

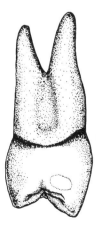

a. General considerations - The distal is remarkably similar to the mesial surface, although it is slightly shorter occlusocervically.

b. Buccal margin - The buccal outline is convex throughout its length, with the crest of curvature in the gingival third.

c. Lingual margin - The lingual margin is almost symmetrical, and is quite convex, especially in the middle third, where the height of contour is located.

d. Occlusal margin - Occlusally, the distal is similar to the mesial aspect, except that the marginal ridge is located at a more cervical level, allowing more of the occlusal surface to be visible. There is normally no marginal groove. In the rare instances when it is present, it is indistinct.

e. Cervical margin - The curvature occlusally is less than on the mesial.

f. Other considerations - The distal contact area is larger than the mesial, and is located at a slightly more cervical level, but still at the junction of the occlusal and middle thirds. Its outline is ovoid, and is wider buccolingually than occlusogingivally.

The distal surface is generally convex in all directions, and does not exhibit the concavity which is present on the mesial surface, although there may sometimes be a flattening in the same area.

7. Occlusal aspect:

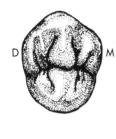

a. General considerations - From the occlusal aspect, the outline of the crown can be described as hexagonal, or six-sided, and it is wider buccolingually than mesiodistally.

b. Buccal outline - The prominent buccal ridge is the primary contributor to the generally convex buccal outline. If the buccal developmental depressions are deep, they may create slight concavities in the outline on either side of the buccal ridge.

c. Lingual margin - The lingual margin is evenly convex, almost in a semi-circle.

d. Mesial and distal margins - The two proximal margins are relatively straight, and they converge toward the lingual. Thus, the lingual portion of the tooth is narrower mesiodistally than the buccal portion. When the mesial marginal groove is prominent, it may create a dip in the mesial outline.

e. Boundaries - The occlusal surface, or occlusal table, is bounded on the mesial and distal by the marginal ridges, and on the buccal and lingual by the mesial and distal cusp ridges of the buccal and lingual cusps.

8. Components of the Occlusal Table:

a. Cusps - There are two cusps, named by location, buccal and lingual. The buccal cusp is normally sharper, longer, and bulkier.

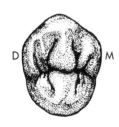

i. Buccal cusp - The buccal cusp tip is located well toward the buccal, and is offset to the distal. It is wider and higher than the lingual cusp.

The buccal cusp has four cusp ridges, and they are named according to the direction they extend from the cusp tip:

Buccal cusp ridge - The buccal cusp ridge extends cervically from the cusp tip on the buccal surface, and corresponds to the previously described buccal ridge.

Lingual cusp ridge - It extends lingually from the cusp tip to the central groove. This cusp ridge is also one of two triangular ridges found on the tooth, so it can be said that the lingual cusp ridge of the buccal cusp is synonymous with the buccal triangular ridge of the tooth. In addition, it may be called the buccal portion of the transverse ridge.

Mesial cusp ridge - The mesial cusp ridge extends mesially from the cusp tip to the mesiobucco-occlusal point angle area.

Distal cusp ridge - It extends distally from the cusp tip to the distobucco-occlusal point angle area. The mesial and distal cusp ridges correspond to the mesio-occlusal and disto-occlusal slopes, which compose the occlusal outline, when the tooth is viewed from the buccal aspect.

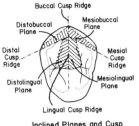

Inclined Planes and Cusp
Ridges of a Buccal Cusp (premolar)

The buccal cusp has four inclined planes, which are the sloping areas located between two adjacent cusp ridges. They take the name of the two cusp ridges which they lie between, as follows:

Mesiobuccal inclined plane
(non-functional)

Distobuccal inclined plane
(non-functional)

Mesiolingual inclined plane
(functional)

Distolingual inclined plane
(functional)

In active occlusion, the buccal cusps of the maxillary posterior teeth are functional only on their lingual side. Hence, the only functional inclined planes of the buccal cusp are those on the lingual, the mesiolingual and the distolingual.

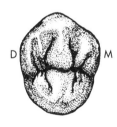

ii. Lingual cusp - The lingual cusp tip is located well to the lingual, and is offset toward the mesial. It is generally smaller and rounder than the buccal cusp. It is the shortest of all the maxillary premolar cusps. It also has four cusp ridges and four inclined planes, which are located and named in the same manner as those of the buccal cusp. Since the lingual cusp is in function on both buccal and lingual sides, it would seem that all four of its inclined planes would be functional. However, as will be pointed out in the next unit, the entire lingual cusp of the mandibular first premolar is normally non-functional. This means that because of the normal manner by which the first premolars of the two arches occlude, the mesiolingual inclined plane of the lingual cusp of the maxillary first premolar is not in function. Therefore, this tooth has only three functional inclined planes associated with its lingual cusp rather than the expected four.

b. Transverse ridge - The buccal and lingual triangular ridges of the tooth meet in the area of the central groove, thus forming a transverse ridge.

c. Marginal ridges - Unlike the marginal ridges of anterior teeth, those of posterior teeth form the mesial and distal borders of the occlusal surface. They are linear ridges which run from the bucco-occlusal point angle to the linguo-occlusal point angle, and are named mesial and distal marginal ridges by their location. The mesial marginal ridge is normally slightly shorter, and its continuity is interrupted by the mesial marginal groove near its midpoint.

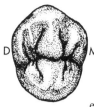

d. Fossae - Fossae are the general depressed areas on the occlusal surfaces of posterior teeth, and the maxillary premolars normally display two of them.

    i. Mesial triangular fossa - This fossa is roughly triangular in shape, and is bounded by the mesial marginal ridge, the transverse ridge, and the mesial cusp ridges of the two cusps.

    ii. Distal triangular fossa - It has a shape and boundaries which are similar to those of the mesial triangular fossa, although it is not quite so deep.

e. Pits and Grooves:

The occlusal surface of the maxillary first premolar normally exhibits two pits, which are located in the deepest portion of the two fossae. They are named by location:

    i. Mesial pit - The mesial pit is located in the mesial triangular fossa just inside the mesial marginal ridge about midway buccolingually.

The mesial pit is the point of union of four primary or developmental grooves:

Mesiolingual triangular groove - This groove extends a short distance from the mesial pit in a mesiolingual direction, where it fades out.

Mesiobuccal triangular groove - It is similar to the ML triangular groove, except that it runs in a mesiobuccal direction.

Central groove - The central groove has a mesiodistal direction and connects the mesial pit and the distal pit.

Mesial marginal groove - The mesial marginal groove extends from the mesial pit in a mesial direction, crossing over the marginal ridge a short distance onto the mesial surface, where it fades out.

    ii. Distal pit - The distal pit is located just inside the distal marginal ridge, midway buccolingually, and is the point of union of three primary grooves:

        DB triangular groove

        DL triangular groove

        Central groove

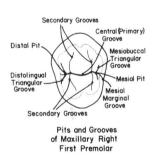

Pits and Grooves
of Maxillary Right
First Premolar

Note: All the grooves described are primary or developmental grooves. Other grooves are sometimes present, as well, and they are normally not given a specific name. They are simply known as supplemental or secondary grooves. On this tooth, the most consistent and easily observable secondary grooves are those which outline the triangular ridges on their mesial and distal borders. This is true of other posterior teeth as well. The maxillary first premolar normally has less secondary grooves than the second premolar.

76

9. Root:

The root structure of the maxillary first premolar is unique among premolars, since there are two branches in a majority of cases, while all other premolars are normally single rooted. Even though two roots are most commonly found in this tooth, there are three identifiable root types, as follows:

a. Type I - Single root:

The single root is quite straight, and tapers fairly evenly from the cervical line to an apex which is rather blunt. It is wider buccolingually than mesiodistally. Both buccal and lingual surfaces are convex, and the buccal portion of the root is slightly wider than the lingual.

The mesial concavity of the crown is usually continuous with a concavity forming a longitudinal groove, or root concavity on the mesial surface of the root. A longitudinal groove is often found on the distal surface as well, but it is not normally as pronounced. Therefore, both mesial and distal surfaces are normally concave, but the mesial surface is much more so.

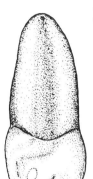

In cross section at mid root, the outline is most often somewhat kidney shaped. The buccal and lingual outlines are convex, but the mesial surface is quite indented, reflecting the mesial root concavity. The distal surface is flat to slightly concave.

TYPE I

b. Type II - Bifurcated root:

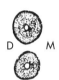

The root trunk divides into a buccal and a lingual root branch. Root trunk is defined as that portion of the root situated between the cervical line and the point of furcation (branching). Thus, a root trunk is found only in multirooted teeth. A type II root is usually bifurcated for at least half its length.

All surfaces of both root branches are convex, and taper to apices which are sharp. The buccal root branch is normally larger in general size, although the two roots are about equal in length.

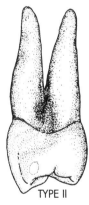

In cross section at the mid root level, both branches are more or less round in outline, with the buccal root outline slightly greater in circumference.

This is the most common root form of maxillary first premolars.

TYPE II

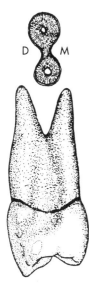

c. Type III - Laminated root:

This type resembles Type II, except the buccal and lingual branches are joined wholly, or in part, by a lamination, which is defined as a thin connection between the main portions of the root structure.

Many variations of the laminated type may be found. The typical hourglass outline of a mid root cross section is similar in all respects to that of the single root, except for the distal outline which is greatly indented, or concave, like the mesial outline, thus leaving a thin connection, or lamination, between the two portions.

TYPE III

10. Variations and anomalies:

a. Crown form generally does not differ widely, although the mesial concavity exhibits considerable variability in its area and depth.

b. Root form is variable, as evidenced by the three common types. Deflected roots and abnormal curvatures are fairly common. Occasionally, a three rooted specimen is found, with two buccal branches, and one lingual branch.

c. The root(s) may, on rare occasions, penetrate the anterior portion of the maxillary sinus, also known as the antrum.

C. The Permanent Maxillary Second Premolar:

1. General characteristics:

a. Arch position - The permanent maxillary second premolar is the fifth tooth from the midline. It shares a mesial contact with the maxillary first premolar and a distal contact with the maxillary first molar. It is a succedaneous tooth, replacing the deciduous maxillary second molar.

b. Universal number:

Maxillary right second premolar - #4

Maxillary left second premolar - #13

c. General form and function - The two maxillary premolars are functionally alike. Structurally, the second premolar closely resembles the first premolar, with some general exceptions:

i. The crown of the second premolar is slightly smaller in all dimensions than that of the first premolar.

ii. The second premolar is generally less blocky, thus exhibiting a more rounded crown form.

iii. The buccal and lingual cusps are of nearly equal height in the second premolar.

iv. There is normally no mesial concavity or marginal groove found on the crown of the second premolar.

v. The second premolar is normally a single rooted tooth.

vi. More variations from normal are observed with second premolar specimens.

2. Development Table: (Maxillary second premolar)*

Initiation of calcification .... 2 to 2 1/4 years

Completion of enamel .... 6 to 7 years

Eruption .... 11 to 12 years

Completion of root .... 12 to 14 years

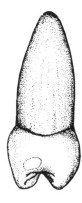

3. Buccal aspect:

The buccal aspect is similar to that of the maxillary first premolar, with the following exceptions:

a. The buccal cusp of the second premolar is not as long or pointed.

b. The cusp tip is offset to the mesial, thus the mesio-occlusal slope is slightly shorter than the disto-occlusal slope. The reverse is true of the first premolar.

c. The mesio-occlusal and disto-occlusal line angles are not as prominent, and the mesial outline is not quite so concave.

4. Lingual aspect:

The lingual aspect is similar to that of the maxillary first premolar, with the following exceptions:

a. The lingual cusp is relatively longer, making the crown longer on the lingual side, and so less of the occlusal surface is visible from this aspect.

b. The lingual cusp tip is not quite so far offset to the mesial.

5. Mesial aspect:

The mesial aspect is similar to the mesial of the maxillary first premolar, with the following exceptions:

a. The two cusps are nearly the same length.

b. There is no mesial concavity, and instead this portion of the crown is slightly flattened or convex.

c. A mesial marginal groove is usually absent.

d. Both the contact area and marginal ridge are located at a slightly more cervical level than on the mesial of the first premolar.

*From Wheeler, R.C.: *Dental Anatomy, Physiology and Occlusion* (5th ed.; Philadelphia: W.B. Saunders Company, 1974).

6. Distal aspect:

The distal aspect is similar to that of the maxillary first premolar, with the following exceptions:

    a. The two cusps are approximately the same length.

    b. The contact area is slightly larger in size, when compared to the first premolar, since the second premolar's distal contact is with the first molar.

    c. Both the distal contact area and marginal ridge are found at a slightly more cervical level than on the distal of the first premolar.

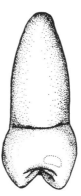

7. Occlusal aspect:

The occlusal aspect differs from the maxillary first premolar in the following ways:

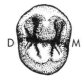

    a. The line angles of the crown are more rounded, and consequently the crown appears less angular. This makes the hexagonal outline more difficult to visualize.

    b. The central groove is often shorter, and may be more irregular, sometimes displaying multiple supplemental grooves. Because of the shorter central groove, the mesial and distal pits are located closer to each other and more to the middle of the occlusal table.

    c. The mesial marginal groove is normally absent, but even if present, it is quite indistinct.

    d. The lingual cusp tip is normally not quite as far offset to the mesial.

    e. On the lingual cusp, there are four functional inclined planes, whereas the first premolar exhibited only three.

8. Root:

    a. The root is normally single, and tapers rather evenly from the cervical line to a relatively blunt apex.

    b. Root length is normally as great, or slightly greater, than the root structure of the first premolar.

    c. The root is wider buccolingually than mesiodistally, with the buccal portion slightly wider mesiodistally than the lingual. Buccal and lingual surfaces are convex, and mesial and distal surfaces are either convex or flat.

d. In cross section views, the root outline is normally ovoid, or a flattened ovoid, wider buccolingually.

e. It is often deflected slightly to the distal in its apical portion.

9. Variations and anomalies:

a. Crown form varies more than in the first premolar. A central groove may be absent, so that only one centrally located pit is present on the occlusal surface.

b. Root variations occur, and distal deflections of the apical third are not uncommon. On occasion, there are two roots, buccally and lingually positioned, similar to those of the type II first premolar.

c. As with the other maxillary posterior teeth, the root occasionally penetrates the antrum.

Maxillary Right First Premolar

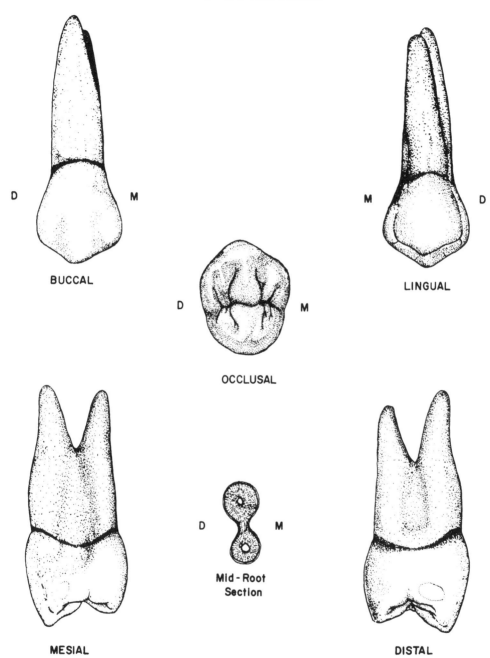

BUCCAL

D M

OCCLUSAL

D M

LINGUAL

M D

MESIAL

D M

Mid - Root
Section

DISTAL

Maxillary First Premolar
Root Variations
Mesial View

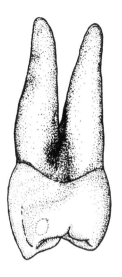

Bifurcated

Mid-Root Section

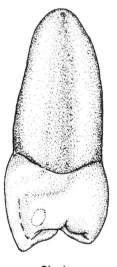

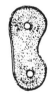

Single

Mid-Root Section

Maxillary Right Second Premolar

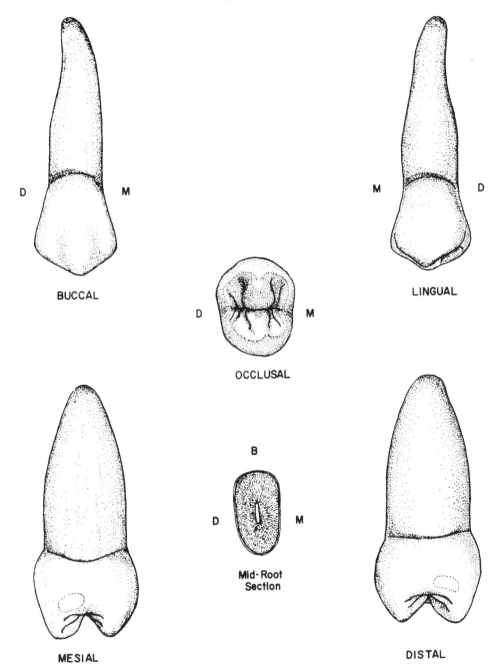

BUCCAL

OCCLUSAL

LINGUAL

B

D M

Mid-Root
Section

MESIAL

DISTAL

84

UNIT # 6

I. **Reading Assignment:**

Unit # 6 (The Permanent Mandibular Premolars)

II. **Specific Objectives:**

At the completion of this unit, the student will be able to:

A. List the appropriate age(s) concerning developmental chronology of the mandibular premolars found in the development tables, or select the appropriate age(s) from a list, when given a certain developmental feature. The student should also be able to compare these ages between the mandibular premolars.

B. Demonstrate a knowledge of the morphology of each surface of the crown, as well as the root, of each permanent mandibular premolar by:

    1. describing,

    2. selecting the correct information from a list,

    3. or interpreting a diagram to identify or name any of the following features:

        a. Contours of any surface or margin of any surface.

        b. Structural entities such as grooves, pits, ridges, inclined planes, cusps, fossae, lobes etc.

        c. Height of contour and contact areas.

        d. Relative dimensions and shape.

        e. Any other surface feature.

Furthermore, the student will be able to make comparisons of any of these features between the mandibular premolars.

C. Make comparisons between mandibular premolars, and other permanent teeth, where appropriate, by selecting the correct response from a list.

D. Make comparisons between the general characteristics of the mandibular premolars, including function, arch position, distinguishing features, etc., by describing them, or selecting the correct response from a list, when given the tooth (teeth), or a description of the general characteristic(s).

E. Determine from a diagram or description whether a given mandibular premolar is first or second, or right or left.

F. Determine the correct universal number, or Palmer notation, for a given diagram or description of any mandibular premolar.

G. Demonstrate a knowledge of any of the new terms in this unit by defining them, or selecting the correct definition or application thereof from a list, when given the term, or any of its applications.

H. Demonstrate a knowledge of any of the variations or anomalies in this unit by describing them, or selecting the correct response from a list, when given the particular tooth (teeth), the anomaly, or any of its features or applications.

The student is also responsible for any material which was to have been mastered in previous units.

THE PERMANENT MANDIBULAR PREMOLARS

I. **Permanent Mandibular Premolars**

    A. Introduction:

        1. As a review of the distinguishing characteristics of premolars, it will be recalled that:

            a. The mandibular first premolar is smaller in general size than the second premolar.

            b. The mandibular premolars' buccolingual and mesiodistal crown dimensions are approximately equal.

            c. The mandibular premolars may have more than two cusps, and lingual cusps are less prominent than those of the maxillary premolars. The single buccal cusp is always more prominent than any lingual cusp.

            d. When viewed from either proximal, the mandibular premolars' crown profile tilts toward the lingual.

            e. The mandibular premolars are normally single rooted.

        2. The two mandibular premolars do not resemble each other nearly as much as do their maxillary counterparts. They are transitional teeth, with the first premolar reflecting the transition from the canine, and the second premolar showing the change toward the molars. The first premolar has a diminutive lingual cusp which is normally non-functional, so that its morphology and role in mastication parallel those of the canine. The second premolar most often has two lingual cusps, and more closely approximates a small molar in structure and function. The slope of the marginal ridges is also transitional. The first premolar exhibits a slope which is more similar to that of anterior teeth, and the second premolar displays a more horizontal angulation like other posterior teeth.

    B. Permanent Mandibular First Premolar:

        1. General characteristics:

            a. Arch position - The mandibular first premolar is the fourth tooth from the midline in each mandibular quadrant of the permanent dentition. It has a mesial contact with the mandibular canine, and a distal contact with the mandibular second premolar. It is a succedaneous tooth, replacing the deciduous first molar.

            b. Universal number:

                Mandibular right first premolar - #28

                Mandibular left first premolar - #21

            c. General form and function - Although the first premolar has two cusps, like most premolars, only the buccal cusp is functional, thus allying it most closely with the canine.

            From the occlusal aspect, the diamond shaped outline of the first premolar resembles that of the canine. From either the facial or lingual aspects, this tooth exhibits a pentagonal form, while the proximal surfaces are rhomboidal in outline.

            In summary, the mandibular first premolar actually is closer in form and masticatory function to a canine than to the other premolar in the mandibular arch. Only in relative size, and appearance from the facial aspect, does this tooth resemble the adjacent second premolar.

2. Development Table: (Mandibular First Premolar)*

Initiation of calcification .... 1 3/4-2 years

Completion of enamel ....5-6 years

Eruption .... 10-11 years

Completion of root .... 12-13 years

3. Buccal aspect:

a. General considerations - The pentagonal outline from the buccal aspect is similar to the facial form of both the canine and second premolar. The buccal surface itself is convex both occlusogingivally and mesiodistally. The occlusocervical dimension is shorter than that of any anterior tooth, but longer than the teeth posterior to it.

b. Mesial margin - The mesial margin is slightly concave from the contact area to the cervical line. The height of contour, at the contact area, is in the middle third.

c. Distal margin - The distal outline is similar to the mesial margin, only a little shorter.

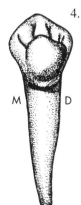

D   M

d. Cervical outline - The cervical line presents an even, slightly convex curve toward the apex. The depth of curvature is less than that of the anterior teeth.

e. Occlusal outline - The pointed buccal cusp tip divides the occlusal outline into two portions, the mesio-occlusal and disto-occlusal slopes, or mesial and distal cusp ridges. The mesio-occlusal slope is normally shorter, thus leaving the cusp tip slightly offset toward the mesial.

f. Other considerations - The buccal ridge, representing the middle buccal lobe, is the most prominent portion of the buccal surface. Mesiobuccal and distobuccal developmental depressions are usually present, but imbrication lines are not normally found.

From this aspect, it is apparent that the contact areas are located at approximately the same level. The marginal ridges display a similar arrangement. This feature is unique to the mandibular first premolar, since on other permanent posterior teeth the distal marginal ridge and contact area are found at a more cervical level. In some specimens of this tooth, the mesial structures are even more cervically located than those on the distal.

The buccal height of contour is found in the cervical third.

4. Lingual aspect:

a. General considerations - The lingual surface lacks the prominent occlusocervical ridge that is present on the facial, and it is consistently convex in all directions. Most of the buccal half of the occlusal table is visible from this aspect, because of the small lingual cusp, and the inclination of the crown toward the lingual. All lingual dimensions are less than those of the buccal surface. The lingual surface is much narrower mesiodistally, due to the lingual convergence of the mesial and distal surfaces. This feature allows a view of most of the mesial and distal surfaces from this aspect.

M   D

---

*From Wheeler, R.C.: *Dental Anatomy, Physiology and Occlusion* (5th ed.; Philadelphia: W.B. Saunders Company, 1974).

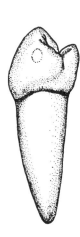

b. Mesial and distal margins - These margins are similar to those of the buccal surface, only much shorter, because the lingual surface itself is shorter.

c. Cervical outline - The CEJ is slightly convex toward the apical.

d. Occlusal outline - The actual occlusal outline is that of the buccal cusp, because of its much greater height. For instructive purposes, however, the outline of the much smaller lingual cusp will be described. The lingual cusp tip is very short, but may be sharp. The disto-occlusal slope is slightly longer than the mesio-occlusal slope, thus the cusp tip is offset to the mesial, like the buccal cusp. Since both cusp tips are mesially offset, the portion of the crown distal to the transverse ridge is larger than the portion mesial to it.

e. Other considerations - The lingual height of contour is located in the middle third.

One of the landmark features of this tooth, and its mesial and lingual aspects in particular, is the mesiolingual developmental groove. This groove originates in the mesial pit of the occlusal surface and crosses onto the mesial surface near the mesiolingual line angle. It normally fades out at about the junction of the cervical and middle thirds. It is visible from this aspect because of the convergence of the mesial surface toward the lingual.

5. Mesial aspect:

a. General considerations - The mesial surface is roughly rhomboidal in form, although this shape is more difficult to visualize than it is on other mandibular posterior teeth, since the lingual outline is so short.

b. Buccal margin - The buccal outline is generally convex, with the height of contour in the gingival third. As is typical of all mandibular posterior teeth, this outline is greatly inclined toward the lingual.

c. Lingual margin - The lingual margin is less convex and much shorter than the buccal outline. The crest of curvature is close to the occlusal limit of the lingual margin, but since the margin is so short, it is in the middle third of the crown.

d. Cervical outline - The cervical line is curved slightly toward the occlusal.

e. Occlusal outline - The occlusal outline reveals the buccal portion of the transverse ridge sloping at approximately a 45° angle, which is nearly paralleled by the outline of the mesial marginal ridge at a more cervical level.

Since the crown profile from this aspect is inclined toward the lingual, the buccal cusp tip is located over the center of the root.

f. Other considerations - The previously described mesiolingual developmental groove is fully visible on the mesial surface near the lingual margin.

The contact area is located toward the buccal, in the middle third. It is circular to somewhat ovoid in shape.

The height of contour of the mesial surface is located in the middle third, in association with the contact area.

6. Distal aspect:

The basic outline and anatomy of the distal surface is similar to the mesial surface, with a few exceptions:

   a. There is no distolingual developmental groove, but there is a <u>distal marginal groove</u>.

   b. The distal surface is a little shorter occlusocervically, and it is wider buccolingually than the mesial surface.

   c. The cervical line curvature is slightly less.

   d. The contact area is similarly shaped, but occupies a slightly broader area, since it approximates the second premolar, which is a larger tooth than the canine. Its location in both dimensions is similar to that of the mesial surface.

   e. The distal marginal ridge does not show quite as steep a slope toward the lingual.

7. Occlusal aspect:

   a. General considerations - From the occlusal aspect, the crown profile is more or less rhomboidal, or diamond shaped, with a notch in the mesial outline at the mesiolingual developmental groove.

   Due to the mesial offset of both cusp tips and thus the transverse ridge, the distal portion of the tooth is larger than the mesial.

   Because of the lingual inclination of the crown of this tooth, much of the buccal surface, but almost none of the lingual surface, may be seen from the occlusal aspect.

   b. Buccal outline - The buccal margin is rather uniformly convex, with well described, though rounded, MB and DB line angles. The outline of the buccal ridge is the most prominent feature of this margin.

   c. Lingual outline - This margin is also convex, but is much shorter than the buccal. Mesially, it ends near the mesiolingual developmental groove.

   d. Mesial outline - The mesial margin is slightly convex to nearly straight. The only exception is the concave offset near the mesiolingual line angle, where the mesiolingual developmental groove traverses it.

   e. Distal outline - The distal outline is more regularly convex than the mesial outline.

   f. Boundaries - The occlusal surface is bounded by the mesial and distal marginal ridges proximally. The boundaries on the buccal and lingual include the mesial and distal cusp ridges of both cusps.

8. Components of the Occlusal Surface:

   a. Cusps - There are two cusps, a buccal and a lingual, with the buccal being much larger and the only functional cusp.

      i. <u>Buccal cusp</u> - The buccal cusp tip is offset to the mesial and located toward the buccal portion of the occlusal surface, but since the crown is so inclined lingually, it is also located approximately over the long axis of the tooth. The cusp has four cusp ridges and four inclined planes, which are named exactly like those of the maxillary premolars. Since this is a mandibular tooth, all four of the inclined planes of the buccal cusp are functional.

      ii. <u>Lingual cusp</u> - The lingual cusp is very small, usually no more than half the height of the buccal cusp. Sometimes it is more of a tubercle than a true cusp. Like the buccal cusp, it is offset to the mesial. It also has four cusp ridges and four inclined planes named like those of the maxillary premolars. Since this cusp itself is normally nonfunctional, none of its inclined planes is considered to be functional.

b. <u>Transverse ridge</u> - As in the maxillary premolars, the buccal and lingual triangular ridges of the tooth meet in the central groove area to form a transverse ridge. The buccal triangular ridge is considerably larger and longer than the lingual, thus comprising a greater portion of the transverse ridge. The central groove, which separates the two component triangular ridges, is sometimes so indistinct in the first premolar, that the two triangular ridges appear to be continuous.

c. Marginal ridges - The <u>mesial marginal ridge</u> slopes from buccal to lingual at a 45° angle, while the marginal ridges of other posterior teeth are roughly horizontal. In fact, it more closely resembles the angulation of the marginal ridges of anterior teeth, especially the canine. The <u>distal marginal ridge</u> is longer, more prominent, and does not exhibit quite as steep a slope toward the lingual.

d. Fossae - The two irregular depressions on the occlusal surface are designated as the <u>mesial</u> and <u>distal fossae</u>. They correspond to the mesial and distal triangular fossae of other posterior teeth, and are bounded by the transverse ridge, the marginal ridges, and the mesial and distal cusp ridges of the two cusps. The mesial fossa is roughly linear in shape, while the distal fossa is larger and more or less circular.

e. Pits and grooves - The two pits on the occlusal surface are found in the deepest portions of the two fossae.

   i. <u>Mesial pit</u> - The mesial pit is located just distal to the mesial marginal ridge, at about the midpoint buccolingually on the occlusal table. It is normally the point of union of three primary grooves.

<u>Central groove</u> - The central groove extends mesiodistally between the two pits.

<u>Mesiobuccal triangular groove</u> - This groove is similar in location to that of the maxillary premolars.

<u>Mesiolingual developmental groove</u> - This unique groove has been previously described from mesial and lingual aspects. On the occlusal surface, it angles mesiolingually from the mesial pit, where it crosses over the mesial marginal ridge onto the mesial surface near the mesiolingual line angle.

On rare occasions, a mesial marginal groove also originates in the mesial pit.

   ii. <u>Distal pit</u> - The distal pit is positioned in the deepest portion of the distal fossa, similar to the location of the mesial pit, and is the junction of four primary grooves:

     <u>Central groove</u>

     <u>Distal marginal groove</u>

     <u>Distolingual triangular groove</u>

     <u>Distobuccal triangular groove</u>

9. Root:

a. The root is normally single, fairly straight, and its outline tapers from the cervical line to a relatively sharp apex.

b. The root length is slightly less than that of the mandibular second premolar, and considerably less than the lower canine.

M D

c. It is wider buccolingually than mesiodistally. The buccal and lingual surfaces are convex, while the mesial and distal surfaces are slightly convex to flat, and converge toward the lingual. Root concavities occur only occasionally.

d. In a midroot cross-section, the outline is roughly ovoid and wider buccolingually than mesiodistally. It is slightly wider at the buccal than at the lingual.

10. Variations and anomalies:

a. The crown of this tooth exhibits wide variation in form. Some of the more common differences include:

i.   An absence of the ML developmental groove.

ii. Two parallel ML developmental grooves.

iii. The size of the lingual cusp, which can range from complete absence to nearly as large as the buccal cusp.

iv. The continuity of the transverse ridge, as it is affected by the depth of the central groove.

v.   The location of the lingual cusp mesiodistally. Although normally slightly offset to the mesial, the lingual cusp tip can be centered mesiodistally, or even offset to the distal.

b. The root, on rare occasions, may display a bifurcation, thus creating buccal and lingual root branches.

C. Permanent Mandibular Second Premolar:

1. General characteristics:

a. Arch position - In the permanent dentition, the mandibular second premolar is the fifth tooth from the midline in each lower quadrant. It has a mesial contact with the mandibular first premolar, and a distal contact with the permanent mandibular first molar. It is the succedaneous tooth for the deciduous mandibular second molar.

b. Universal number:

Mandibular right second premolar - #29

Mandibular left second premolar - #20

c. General form and function - The second premolar has a generally larger crown, and a slightly larger and longer root than the first premolar. The opposite arrangement is true for the crowns of maxillary premolars, where the first premolar is slightly larger.

From the facial aspect, the general shape of the crown is similar to that of the mandibular first premolar. However, from all other aspects, differences are apparent. There are two general forms of the mandibular second premolar, with the most common form exhibiting two lingual cusps, while the other type displays but one. The difference between the two types is primarily in occlusal form, since the other surface contours are similar.

Regardless of the number of lingual cusps, the occlusal table is most similar to that of a small molar. Consequently, this tooth functions in a grinding capacity with the molars, as contrasted to the first premolar which functions much like the canine.

2. Development Table (Mandibular Second Premolar)*

Initiation of calcification .... 2 1/4 to 2 1/2 years

Completion of enamel .... 6 to 7 years

Eruption .... 11 to 12 years

Completion of root .... 13 to 14 years

3. Buccal aspect:

a. The mandibular second premolar resembles the mandibular first premolar from the buccal, with the following exceptions:

i.   The tooth is slightly larger, even though the tip of the buccal cusp is shorter and the occlusocervical dimension is a little less. Since the cusp tip is not so high, it is not as sharp and the mesio-occlusal and disto-occlusal slopes are not as inclined.

ii.   The cusp tip is also centered mesiodistally, making the two slopes approximately equal in length.

Despite these slight differences, it is difficult to distinguish between the two mandibular premolars from this aspect.

b. The location and morphology of the structures of the facial surface, including height of contour, are also similar to those of the first premolar.

4. Lingual aspect:

a. General considerations - The lingual cusp or cusps, are better developed and higher in comparison to the first premolar. The lingual surface is generally smooth and convex.

b. The mesial, distal, and cervical outlines are similar to those of the first premolar, although the lingual surface is considerably wider mesiodistally, and longer occlusocervically.

c. Occlusal outline - The lingual cusps are higher, and as a consequence, much less of the occlusal surface can be seen from this aspect, when compared to the first premolar. The height of the lingual cusp(s) is still somewhat less than the buccal cusp height.

i.   The three cusp type exhibits a mesiolingual and a distolingual cusp. Between the two lingual cusps a lingual groove extends a short distance onto the lingual surface. The mesiolingual cusp is wider and longer, while the distolingual cusp is smaller, but often is the sharper of the two. This arrangement leaves the lingual groove offset to the distal in the occlusal outline.

ii.   The two cusp type displays a single lingual cusp. There is no lingual groove, but a depression is often found toward the distal portion of the surface. The single cusp is approximately the same height as the mesiolingual cusp of the three cusp type.

d. The height of contour of the lingual surface is found in the occlusal third of the crown.

*From Wheeler, *R.C.: Dental Anatomy, Physiology and Occlusion* 5th ed.; Philadelphia: W.B. Saunders Company, 1974).

92

5. Mesial aspect:

From the mesial aspect, the two mandibular premolars are similar, but much easier to differentiate than from the facial aspect. Dimensionally, the second premolar is wider buccolingually, but slightly shorter occlusocervically. Structurally, the two premolars differ in the following ways:

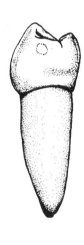

a. The lingual inclination of the crown and of its buccal surface is not quite as great as on the first premolar. Consequently, the buccal cusp tip is not centered over the root, but rather is buccal of center. The buccal cusp tip is also shorter and less sharp.

b. Lingual cusps are more prominent than on the first premolar. In the three cusp type, the DL cusp is not visible from the mesial aspect.

c. Occlusogingivally, the mesial surface is convex in the occlusal portion, and concave in the gingival portion.

d. The contact area is located toward the buccal, at the junction of the occlusal and middle thirds. It is larger in size than the mesial contact of the first premolar. It is also roughly circular in outline.

e. The marginal ridge is more nearly horizontal, and much less of the occlusal surface is visible.

f. The landmark of the first premolar, the mesiolingual developmental groove, is absent on the second premolar, but there is normally a mesial marginal groove present.

g. The height of contour of the lingual margin is found in the occlusal third, a location which is unique to the mandibular second premolar.

h. The cervical line shows less depth in its occlusal curvature.

6. Distal aspect:

The distal surface is similar to the mesial surface, except in the following ways:

a. The distal marginal ridge is more cervically placed than on the mesial, resulting in more of the occlusal surface being visible from this aspect, as well as a shorter surface occlusocervically.

b. In the three cusp type, the tips of both the mesiolingual cusp and the distolingual cusp are visible.

c. The contact area is similarly located, but because it is shared with the first molar, it is larger and somewhat ovoid, wider buccolingually than occlusocervically.

7. Occlusal aspect:

a. General considerations - The general shape of the crown from this aspect is more nearly square especially in the three cusp type, when compared to the first premolar. The convergence of the mesial and distal surfaces toward the lingual is not nearly so severe.

b. General groove pattern - The occlusal groove pattern is responsible for the names of the second premolar types. For example, the main groove pattern on the three cusp type takes the form of a "Y", and it is thus named Y type. The main groove pattern on the two cusp type resembles a "U" or "H", resulting in U type and H type second premolars. The Y type is the most common form of mandibular second premolar, and is present in the majority of cases. The two cusp types are less often seen, with H type specimens more common than U type.

c. Three cusp type - (Y type):

i. General occlusal form - The outline of the Y type from the occlusal aspect is roughly square lingual to the buccal line angles, which are quite distinct. On an occasional specimen, the mesiodistal dimension of the crown is even greater through the lingual line angle area than it is through the buccal portion. The Y pattern of the occlusal table is formed by a combination of the central and lingual grooves.

ii. Cusps - The three cusps vary in height and size from largest to smallest, as follows: buccal cusp, mesiolingual cusp, and distolingual cusp. Each cusp exhibits four cusp ridges and four inclined planes, and they are named like those of other posterior teeth. The buccal cusp has four functional inclined planes, while the lingual cusps possess two functional inclined planes each. There is no transverse ridge on the Y type second premolar.

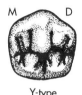

Y-type

iii. Fossae - There are two fossae, the mesial and distal triangular fossae. Both are relatively shallow and irregular, but are more linear in form than the triangular fossae of the maxillary premolars. They are located just inside the marginal ridges, and are also bounded by two cusp ridges of each appropriate cusp. For example, the mesial triangular fossa is bounded by the mesial and lingual cusp ridges of the buccal cusp, and the buccal and mesial cusp ridges of the mesiolingual cusp, in addition to the mesial marginal ridge.

iv. Pits and grooves - There are three pits present on the occlusal table:

Mesial pit - The mesial pit is located in the deepest portion of the mesial triangular fossa, which is about midway from buccal to lingual just inside the mesial marginal ridge. It is the point of union of the following four primary grooves:

Central groove - It extends from the mesial pit to the distal pit in a shallow "V" form.

Mesiolingual triangular groove

Mesiobuccal triangular groove

Mesial marginal groove

Distal pit - Its location in the depth of the distal triangular fossa is similar to that of the mesial pit, and it is also the point of union of four primary grooves:

Central groove

Distolingual triangular groove

Distobuccal triangular groove

Distal marginal groove

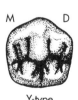

Y-type

Central pit - The central pit is the deepest of the three pits. It is located toward the lingual, and more than halfway from mesial to distal, since the ML cusp is wider than the DL cusp. The central pit is located along the central groove, where it joins the lingual groove, which itself exits the occlusal surface between the two lingual cusps. The central pit is thus the junction of two primary grooves.

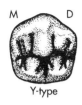

Y-type

Note: Some anatomists prefer to divide the central groove into two grooves as follows:

Mesial groove - The mesial groove extends distolingually from the mesial pit to the central pit.

Distal groove - The distal groove extends mesiolingually from the distal pit to the central pit.

However, this text will consider that there is but one groove, the central groove, with mesial and distal portions, rather than a division into two separate grooves.

d. Two cusp types (U and H types)

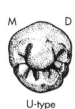

U-type

i. General occlusal form - Two cusp type second premolars exhibit a rounded outline lingual to the buccal line angles, and the buccal line angles are themselves more rounded and less distinct than in the Y type. The mesial and distal surfaces may converge somewhat more toward the lingual, making the lingual portion narrower than the buccal, but the taper is never to the degree of the first premolar. The one lingual cusp is placed directly opposite the buccal cusp and their respective triangular ridges create a transverse ridge. These teeth do not have either a lingual groove or a central pit.

ii. Cusps - The buccal cusp is larger and somewhat higher than the lingual cusp. The lingual cusp sometimes appears as an irregular convexity, rather than a distinct cusp, especially in the U type. The lingual cusp of the H type is larger and sharper than in the U type, and on both types it is offset to the mesial. Both buccal and lingual cusps have four cusp ridges, and four inclined planes, which are named like the same structures on other premolars. The buccal cusp features four functional inclined planes, while the lingual cusp has two.

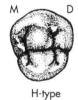

H-type

iii. Fossae - The two cusp type also has two fossae. However, they are roughly circular in shape, and are termed mesial and distal fossa, both facts differing from the three cusp type. They are bounded by the transverse ridge, and appropriate marginal ridges and cusp ridges.

iv. Pits and grooves (U type) - The U pattern is formed by the central groove, portions of the two buccal triangular grooves, and the secondary grooves of the buccal cusp. The central groove extends from the mesial pit to the distal pit, and in the process forms the lower portion of the "U". It can thus be characterized as crescent shaped. The only two pits, the mesial and distal pits, are the point of union of the same four primary grooves previously described in the Y type.

v. Pits and grooves (H type) - The H pattern is formed by the central groove, portions of the four triangular grooves, and the secondary grooves of the buccal and lingual cusps. The central groove runs roughly in a straight line between the two pits, in contrast to the crescent shape of the U type. Pits, fossae, and grooves are named as in the U type.

8. Root:

a. The root is normally single, and tapers evenly to the apex which is relatively sharp. It often has a slight distal inclination in the apical third.

b. The root is slightly wider and longer than that of the first premolar.

c. The general shape of the root from all aspects, as well as in mid root cross section, is similar to that of the first premolar.

9. Variations and anomalies:

   a. In three cusp type crowns, the comparative size of the ML and DL cusps is quite variable. The DL cusp ranges from a barely discernible bump to approximately the same size as the ML cusp.

   b. Anomalies are rare, although a root bifurcation into buccal and lingual branches is sometimes seen.

   c. The mandibular second premolars are, on occasion, congenitally missing. This phenomenon may occur either unilaterally or bilaterally.

   d. Supernumerary teeth are sometimes observed in the mandibular premolar area.

Mandibular Right First Premolar

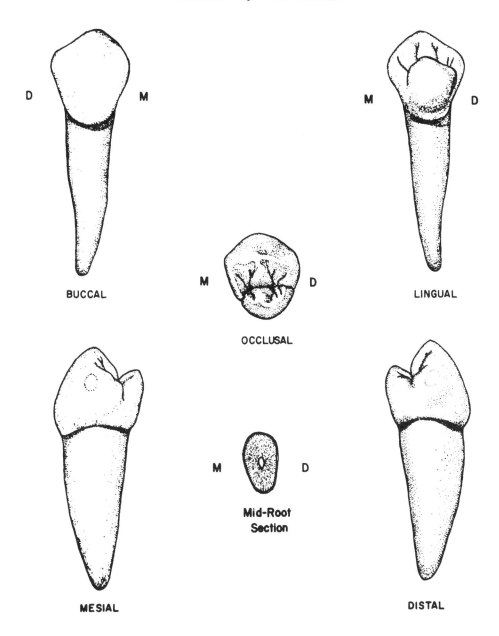

BUCCAL

OCCLUSAL

LINGUAL

Mid-Root
Section

MESIAL

DISTAL

Mandibular Right Second Premolar
(Y-Type Shown In Four Aspects)

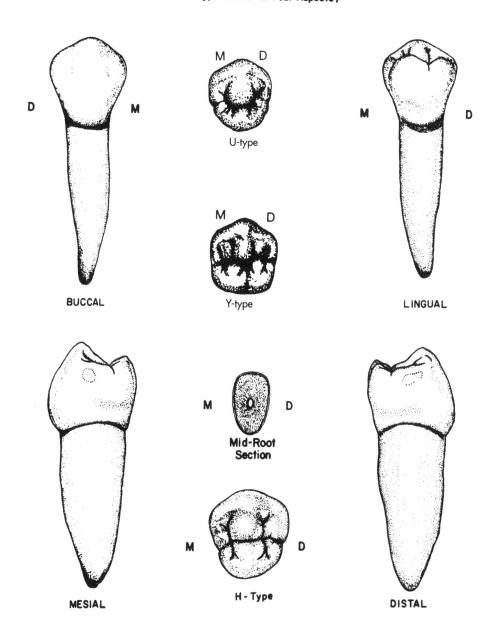

D   M

M   D

M   D
U-type

M   D
Y-type

BUCCAL   LINGUAL

M   D
Mid-Root
Section

M   D
H - Type

MESIAL   DISTAL

UNIT # 7

I. **Reading Assignment:**

Unit # 7 (The Permanent Maxillary Molars)

II. **Specific Objectives:**

At the completion of this unit, the student will be able to:

A. List the appropriate age(s) concerning developmental chronology of the maxillary molars found in the development tables, or select the appropriate age(s) from a list, when given a certain developmental feature. The student should also be able to compare these ages among the maxillary molars.

B. Demonstrate a knowledge of the morphology of each surface of the crown, as well as the root, of each permanent maxillary molar by:

    1. describing,

    2. selecting the correct information from a list,

    3. or interpreting a diagram to identify or name any of the following features:

        a. Contours of any surface, or margin of any surface.

        b. Structural entities such as grooves, pits, ridges, inclined planes, cusps, fossae, lobes, etc.

        c. Height of contour and contact areas.

        d. Relative dimensions and shape.

        e. Any other surface features.

Furthermore, the student will be able to make comparisons of any of the above features among maxillary molars.

C. Make comparisons between permanent maxillary molars and other permanent teeth where appropriate, by selecting the correct response from a list.

D. Make comparisons in the general characteristics of the maxillary molars, including function, arch position, distinguishing features, etc., by describing them, or selecting the correct response from a list when given the tooth (teeth), or a description of the general characteristic(s).

E. Determine from a diagram or description whether a given permanent maxillary molar is first, second, or third, or right or left.

F. Determine the correct universal number or Palmer notation for a given diagram or description of any permanent maxillary molar.

G. Demonstrate a knowledge of any of the new terms in this unit by defining them, or selecting the correct definition, or application thereof, from a list, when given the term, or any of its applications.

H. Demonstrate a knowledge of any of the variations or anomalies in this unit by describing them, or selecting the correct response from a list, when given the particular tooth (teeth), the anomaly, or any of its features or applications.

The student is also responsible for any material which was to have been mastered in previous units.

UNIT # 7
THE PERMANENT MAXILLARY MOLARS

I.   Permanent Molars:

A.   As a group, permanent molars are the largest and most posteriorly located teeth in the mouth. They erupt distal to the deciduous dentition, and hence are not succedaneous. In a normal eruption sequence for permanent teeth, molars are the initial, as well as the final teeth to emerge, with the eruption of all the anterior teeth and premolars sandwiched between.

B.   There are three permanent molars per quadrant, six per arch, and twelve in total. From mesial to distal in each quadrant, they are named permanent <u>first, second</u>, and <u>third molars</u>. The first and second molars are also called <u>six year molars</u>, and <u>twelve year molars</u>, respectively, because of their approximate time of eruption. The third molar, also known as the <u>wisdom tooth</u>, is extremely variable in its time of eruption, as well as its anatomical form. Third molars exhibit a wide range of crown shapes, sizes, contours, and root numbers and forms.

C.   Just as the permanent canines are considered to be the cornerstones of each arch in position, form, and function, the permanent first molars are thought of as cornerstones in the development of occlusion. This is due to their early eruption date, and location in the arch, compared to the other teeth of both dentitions. This topic will be more fully explored later in the text.

D. The molars' function in mastication is mainly grinding. They are ideally designed and situated to accomplish this role. They also function in esthetics and phonetics, but to a more limited extent than the teeth anterior to them. Nevertheless, their contribution to esthetics through muscle support and maintenance of the vertical dimension is important.

E.   There are several factors which aid in distinguishing molars from other permanent teeth:

   1.   Their crowns are generally the largest and most complex.

   2.   Their crowns normally exhibit at least 3 cusps, and usually more, of which at least two are buccal cusps.

   3.   They are normally multirooted.

II.   Permanent Maxillary Molars:

A.   Introduction:

The maxillary molars are the largest teeth in the maxillary arch. Their crown is usually shorter occlusogingivally than the crowns of the teeth anterior to them, but it is much larger in all other measurements. Normally, the first molar is the largest in size, and the second and third molars are progressively smaller.

B.   Features of maxillary molars which aid in differentiating them from other permanent teeth, particularly mandibular molars, include:

   1.   Crowns which are wider buccolingually than mesiodistally. Mandibular molars are wider in the mesiodistal dimension.

   2.   The presence of four cusps in most specimens, of which the size of the two lingual cusps differs greatly. Some mandibular molars display four cusps, but the two lingual cusps are approximately equal in size.

   3.   The presence of an oblique ridge and a distolingual groove on the occlusal surface. No comparable structures are found on the mandibular molars.

   4.   Crowns which are rhomboidal or heart-shaped from the occlusal aspect. Mandibular molars exhibit a rectangular or pentagonal outline from this aspect.

5.   Crowns which are trapezoidal in outline from the mesial or distal aspect. Mandibular molars are rhomboidal and inclined to the lingual in a proximal view.

6.   The presence of three root branches in most cases. Mandibular molars normally exhibit two roots.

C.   Permanent Maxillary First Molar:

1.   General characteristics:

a.   Arch position - The permanent maxillary first molar is the sixth tooth from the midline in each maxillary quadrant. It has a mesial contact with the second deciduous molar, until that tooth is exfoliated. The mesial contact is then shared with the permanent second premolar when it erupts at about age 12. There is no distal contact until the permanent second molar erupts sometime around the age of 12. Permanent molars do not replace deciduous teeth, hence are not succedaneous.

b.   Universal number:

Maxillary right first molar - #3

Maxillary left first molar - #14

c.   General form and function - The maxillary first molar is the largest tooth in the maxillary arch, and in fact, has the largest crown in the mouth. It is much more complex than the maxillary premolars in both crown and root form. Of all the maxillary molars, the first molar is the least variable in anatomic form, and is thus the standard to which the other maxillary molars are compared.

The crown is wider buccolingually than mesiodistally. It is shorter occlusogingivally than the maxillary premolars, the only dimension in which it is less. All four vertical crown surfaces exhibit a trapezoidal outline. The occlusal aspect is similarly foursided, but in a unique, rhomboidal configuration.

Normally, there are three roots, two buccally located, and one lingually placed.

As with all the molars, the main masticatory function is grinding.

2.   Development Table: (Maxillary First Molar)*

Initiation of calcification .... at birth

Completion of enamel .... 3 to 4 years

Eruption .... 6 to 7 years

Completion of root .... 9 to 10 years

3.   Buccal aspect:

a.   General considerations - From the buccal aspect, the general shape of the tooth is trapezoidal, with the longer parallel side at the occlusal. The buccal surface is much larger than that of the premolars, despite the fact that the occlusogingival dimension is slightly less. Because of the rhomboidal crown form, a portion of the distal surface is visible from this aspect. Also visible are the tips of all the major cusps, except the distolingual.

*From Wheeler, R.C.: *Dental Anatomy, Physiology and Occlusion* (5th ed.; Philadelphia: W.B. Saunders Company, 1974).

b. Mesial outline - The mesial outline is flat from the cervical margin occlusally to the contact area, which is the height of contour, and is located at the junction of the occlusal and middle thirds. Occlusally from the contact area, the mesial margin is convex, and joins the occlusal margin in a slightly rounded, but well defined mesio-occlusal angle.

c. Distal outline - The entire distal outline is convex occlusogingivally, with the height of contour associated with the contact area in the middle third. The disto-occlusal angle is more rounded than the mesio-occlusal angle.

d. Cervical outline - The cervical line is slightly and irregularly curved apically with much less curvature than is found in anterior teeth or premolars. However, there may be a sharp dip, or point, in this margin, just occlusal to the furcation area.

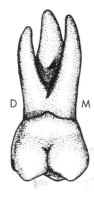

e. Occlusal outline - The occlusal margin is divided into two parts by the concavity of the buccal groove. These two portions outline the two buccal cusps, the mesiobuccal cusp and the distobuccal cusp. The outline of the mesiobuccal cusp is wider, but the distobuccal cusp tip is sharper. The two buccal cusps are approximately the same height, and the mesiolingual cusp tip is visible between them.

f. Other considerations - In the occlusal portion of the buccal surface, the buccal groove occupies a shallow occlusogingival concavity, which extends apically about halfway to the cervical margin. There it most often fades out, but it may end in a buccal pit, or terminate by splitting into two slanting grooves, which extend a short distance before fading out.

The buccal ridges of the two buccal cusps are convex areas on the buccal surface which extend cervically about half its length. They lie on either side of the occlusocervical concavity containing the buccal groove.

In a limited number of specimens, a buccogingival (buccocervical) ridge is found. It is a convexity which extends horizontally, from mesial to distal, in the entire cervical third of the buccal surface, but is most prominent in the mesial portion.

There may be a shallow concavity which extends mesiodistally in the middle third of the surface. When present, it is located just cervical to the buccal ridges, and includes the termination area of the buccal groove.

The height of contour of the buccal surface is located in the cervical third.

4. Lingual aspect:

a. General considerations - The lingual surface is about as wide mesiodistally as the buccal surface, and it is also trapezoidal. The lingual surface shows a more general convexity occlusogingivally than does the buccal surface.

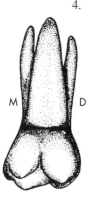

b. Mesial outline - The mesial outline is similar to the buccal aspect.

c. Distal outline - The distal margin is also similar to the buccal aspect, except it is shorter and the disto-occlusal angle is more rounded, since the DL cusp is much smaller than the DB cusp.

d. Cervical outline - The CEJ is slightly and irregularly convex toward the apex.

102

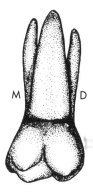

M D

e. Occlusal margin - As on the buccal surface, a groove (the distolingual groove) separates the occlusal margin into two unequal portions. The mesiolingual cusp outline is much longer and larger, but blunter than the outline of the distolingual cusp. In fact, the mesiolingual cusp is normally the largest and longest cusp on this tooth.

f. Other considerations - The distolingual groove originates on the occlusal surface, and crosses onto the lingual surface distal to the midpoint of the occlusal outline. After slanting mesially and cervically, it normally terminates in a lingual pit but may simply fade out. The termination is at a point which is approximately the middle of the lingual surface.

The lingual ridges of the two lingual cusps lie mesial and distal to the concavity containing the distolingual groove. The lingual ridge of the mesiolingual cusp is much the larger and bulkier of the two.

Arising from the lingual portion of the mesiolingual cusp is a tubercle or minicusp that is known as the cusp of Carabelli. A groove normally separates the cusp of Carabelli from the mesiolingual cusp, and is appropriately named the cusp of Carabelli groove. The prominence of the cusp of Carabelli and its accompanying groove varies greatly from tooth to tooth, but most specimens show at least a trace of the trait.

The height of contour is located in the middle third of the lingual surface.

5. Mesial aspect:

a. General considerations - The mesial surface exhibits a roughly trapezoidal shape that is wider at the cervical than at the occlusal, which is the reverse of the buccal and lingual surfaces.

b. Buccal margin - Beginning at the cervical line, the buccal outline is convex in the cervical third, especially so if there is a buccogingival ridge. Then it is flat to slightly concave for a short distance in the middle third. From this point to the cusp tip, the outline is straight, or slightly convex. The height of contour is in the gingival third.

c. Lingual margin - The lingual outline is convex throughout its length, but may be irregular if the cusp of Carabelli is prominent. The height of contour is located in the middle third.

d. Cervical margin - The cervical line is shallow, and irregularly curved toward the occlusal.

e. Occlusal margin - The only cusps which are visible are the two mesial cusps. The outline of the mesial marginal ridge curves irregularly toward the cervical line. There is normally a mesial marginal groove notching the marginal ridge outline about midway along its length.

f. Other considerations - The mesial surface is wider at the cervical than at the occlusal, due to the general convergence of both the buccal and lingual surfaces toward the occlusal.

The contact area varies from round to somewhat ovoid, and is situated slightly to the buccal, at the junction of the occlusal and middle thirds.

The occlusal half of the surface is convex, but there is usually a buccolingual flattening, or even a slight concavity, located cervical to the contact area.

103

6. Distal aspect:

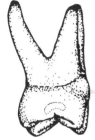

a. General considerations - The distal resembles the mesial surface, but with slightly lessened dimensions. The trapezoidal outline is not as pronounced either, because on the distal surface the cervical width is more nearly equal to the occlusal width.

b. Buccal, lingual, and cervical outlines - All of these outlines are similar to their description for the mesial aspect.

c. Occlusal outline - The mesial cusp tips are visible projecting beyond the outline of the distal cusps. The distal marginal ridge is less prominent and dips farther cervically than on the mesial, thus allowing more of the occlusal surface to be seen. There is usually a distal marginal groove situated about midway along its extent.

d. Cervical outline - The cervical line reveals very little curvature occlusally, and may approach a straight line in some specimens.

e. Other considerations - Because of the crown's rhomboidal shape, much of the buccal surface can be seen from the distal.

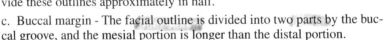

The distal contact area is larger than the mesial contact area, and irregularly long buccolingually, and narrow occlusogingivally. It is located in the middle third, about midway between the buccal and lingual margins.

There may be a slight flattening or concavity in the cervical third, but when present it is never as pronounced as on the mesial.

7. Occlusal aspect:

a. General form - From the occlusal aspect, this tooth has a novel rhomboidal form. This shape creates mesiobuccal and distolingual line angles which are acute, and mesiolingual and distobuccal line angles that are obtuse. The outline is wider buccolingually than mesiodistally, although these dimensions are more nearly equal than in any of the other maxillary posterior teeth.

b. Mesial and distal outlines - The mesial and distal marginal grooves divide these outlines approximately in half.

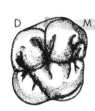

c. Buccal margin - The facial outline is divided into two parts by the buccal groove, and the mesial portion is longer than the distal portion.

d. Lingual margin - The lingual margin is also divided into two convex portions by the distolingual groove, and the mesial portion is longer and less convex than the distal portion.

e. Boundaries - The occlusal table is bounded mesially and distally by the marginal ridges, and on the buccal and lingual by the mesial and distal cusp ridges of the four major cusps.

8. Components of the Occlusal Table:

a. Cusps - There are four major cusps and one minor, sometimes indistinct cusp, which is the cusp of Carabelli.

   i. Mesiobuccal cusp - It is quite sharp, and the second largest in size. Its four cusp ridges are named according to the direction they extend from the cusp tip similar to those of other posterior teeth. They are described anatomically as follows:

   Buccal cusp ridge - The buccal cusp ridge extends from the cusp tip about halfway toward the cervical margin on the buccal surface.

   Lingual cusp ridge - It extends lingually from the cusp tip to the mesial portion of the central groove, where it meets the buccal cusp ridge of the

ML cusp to form a transverse ridge. It is also known as the triangular ridge of the MB cusp.

Mesial cusp ridge - The mesial cusp ridge extends from the cusp tip mesially to the mesiobucco-occlusal point angle.

Distal cusp ridge - It extends from the cusp tip distally to the buccal groove.

Inclined planes - The MB cusp has four inclined planes. The two that are functional are associated with the lingual ridge of the cusp, and are named the mesiolingual and distolingual inclined planes.

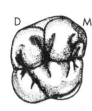

ii. Distobuccal cusp - The DB cusp is the sharpest and third largest of the four major cusps. The cusp ridges and inclined planes are named similarly to those of the MB cusp and only the two lingual inclined planes are functional. Its lingual cusp ridge or triangular ridge forms the buccal portion of the oblique ridge of the tooth.

iii. Mesiolingual cusp - The ML cusp is the largest cusp, but its tip is rounded and blunt. The cusp ridges are similar to those of the other cusps, except the distal cusp ridge. It extends from the ML cusp tip in a distobuccal direction, where it meets the lingual cusp ridge of the DB cusp to form an oblique ridge. The distal cusp ridge is the fifth triangular ridge on the occlusal table, and is thus the only triangular ridge which is not a buccal or lingual cusp ridge. In addition, the buccal cusp ridge forms the lingual portion of the transverse ridge. All four of the ML cusp's inclined planes are functional.

iv. Distolingual cusp - The DL cusp is the smallest and most variable of the four major cusps. Its four cusp ridges and four functional inclined planes are similar to those of other posterior teeth although the buccal cusp ridge extends mesiobucally and the distal cusp ridge extends distobuccally.

v. Cusp of Carabelli - The cusp of Carabelli has been previously discussed.

b. Transverse ridge - The buccal cusp ridge of the mesiolingual cusp and lingual cusp ridge of the mesiobuccal cusp form a transverse ridge.

c. Oblique ridge - An oblique ridge is created by the union of the distal cusp ridge of the mesiolingual cusp and the lingual cusp ridge of the distobuccal cusp.

d. Marginal ridges - The two marginal ridges are named mesial and distal marginal ridges like those of other posterior teeth. They enclose the occlusal surface at these two margins. The mesial marginal ridge is longer and more prominent.

e. Fossae - There are four fossae, and they are named as follows:

i. Central fossa - The central fossa is roughly triangular in shape, and located mesial to the oblique ridge and distal to the transverse ridge in the central portion of the occlusal table. It is bounded by the mesial cusp ridge of the DB cusp, the distal cusp ridge of the MB cusp, the oblique ridge, and the transverse ridge. The central fossa is the largest and deepest of the four fossae.

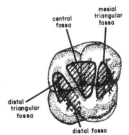

central fossa

mesial triangular fossa

distal triangular fossa

distal fossa

ii. <u>Distal fossa</u> - The distal fossa is more or less linear in shape, and located directly distal and parallel to the oblique ridge. It is continuous with the distal triangular fossa in its distobuccal portion, and is otherwise bounded by the oblique ridge on the mesial, and the mesial and distal cusp ridges of the DL cusp on the distal.

iii. <u>Mesial triangular fossa</u> - This fossa is triangular in shape, and is located just distal to the mesial marginal ridge. It is bounded by the mesial marginal ridge, the transverse ridge, and the mesial cusp ridges of the MB and ML cusps.

iv. <u>Distal triangular fossa</u> - This fossa is also triangular in shape, and is located just mesial to the distal marginal ridge. It is continuous with the distal fossa in its mesial portion, and is bounded on the distal by the distal marginal ridge.

f. Pits and Grooves:

i. <u>Central pit</u> - The central pit is located in the deepest portion of the central fossa at about the center of the occlusal surface. This pit is the junction of two primary developmental grooves:

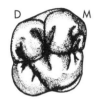

<u>Buccal groove</u> - The buccal groove extends from the central pit in a buccal direction until it passes onto the buccal surface.

<u>Central groove</u> - The central groove extends in a mesiodistal direction connecting the mesial and distal pits. It is composed of a <u>mesial portion</u> which extends mesially from the central pit to the mesial pit, and a <u>distal portion</u> which passes distolingually from the central pit, where it crosses the oblique ridge, to the distal pit.

ii. <u>Mesial pit</u> - The mesial pit is located halfway buccolingually, and just distal to the mesial marginal ridge in the deepest portion of the mesial triangular fossa. It is the junction of four primary developmental grooves.

<u>Central groove</u> (mesial portion) - This groove has been previously described.

<u>Mesiobuccal triangular groove</u> - This groove extends a short distance from the pit toward the mesiobuccal line angle where it fades out.

<u>Mesiolingual triangular groove</u> - This groove extends from the pit toward the mesiolingual line angle a short distance where it fades out.

<u>Mesial marginal groove</u> - It extends mesially over the marginal ridge onto the mesial surface.

iii. <u>Distal pit</u> - The distal pit is located midway buccolingually, and just mesial to the distal marginal ridge. Because the distal pit is located in the area where the distal fossa and distal triangular fossa are confluent, it is a component of both of them. It is the junction of five primary developmental grooves:

<u>Central groove</u> (Distal portion) - This groove has been previously described.

<u>Distolingual groove</u> - The DL groove extends obliquely onto the lingual surface, paralleling the oblique ridge to its distal.

<u>Distobuccal triangular groove</u> - This groove extends a short distance from the distal pit toward the distobuccal line angle, where it fades out.

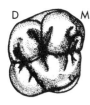

Distolingual triangular groove - It extends a short distance from the distal pit toward the distolingual line angle, where it fades out.

Distal marginal groove - The distal marginal groove extends distally from the distal marginal ridge onto the distal surface.

Roots:

a. The root trunk trifurcates into three well developed root branches, which are named by their location. The two buccal roots are termed mesiobuccal and distobuccal roots, while the one root at the lingual is termed simply, the lingual root.

    i. Lingual root - This root is the largest, longest, and strongest of the three roots. It inclines mostly in a lingual direction from the trifurcation. It is wider mesiodistally than buccolingually, a feature which is unique to this root. From the buccal aspect, it is visible between the two buccal roots, and the apex is normally located almost directly under the buccal groove.

    ii. Mesiobuccal root - The MB root is the second largest and longest of the roots. It inclines mesially and buccally to the apical third, where it curves distally. It is thicker buccolingually, than mesiodistally, and it has a somewhat blunted apex.

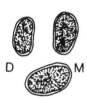

    iii. Distobuccal root - The DB root is the smallest, shortest, and weakest branch. It inclines distally and buccally to the apical third, where it curves mesially. It is a little thicker buccolingually than mesiodistally, and tapers to a fairly sharp apex.

    iv. Mid root section - In cross section at the midroot level, the root outlines of all three branches are roughly ovoid. The two buccal roots are wider buccolingually, while the lingual root is wider mesiodistally. The lingual root outline is generally the largest, followed closely by the MB root outline, while the outline of the DB root is the smallest.

10. Variations and anomalies:

a. For the most part, crown variations are slight. However, the cusp of Carabelli varies greatly in prominence, and is well defined in something less than half the first molars. Even though there may not be much of a cusp, there is usually at least a trace of the cusp of Carabelli groove in almost all specimens, unless attrition has obliterated it.

b. A sharp projection of enamel into the bifurcation area on the facial surface is a variation found in 17% of the maxillary molars, according to one study. This feature affects the curvature of the cervical line, and may be a factor in periodontal disease in this area.

c. The mulberry molar, which is the posterior counterpart of Hutchinson's incisor, due to the similar etiology of congenital syphilis, is occasionally found. The cusps of the mulberry molar are more centrally located than in the normal molar, and the occlusal enamel appears gnarled.

d. Root variations are most often manifest in partial fusion of the root branches, especially of the buccal roots, and by abnormal lengths and curvatures.

e. As with other maxillary posterior teeth, root branches of the first molar may penetrate the maxillary sinus.

D. Permanent Maxillary Second Molar:

1. General characteristics:

a. Arch position - The maxillary second molar is the seventh tooth and second molar from the midline, in each upper quadrant of the permanent dentition. It has a mesial contact with the permanent first molar, and a distal contact with the permanent third molar, if and when that tooth erupts. It is not a succedaneous tooth.

b. Universal number:

Maxillary right second molar - #2

Maxillary left second molar - #15

c. General form and function - The crown is similar in form to the maxillary first molar, but is generally smaller, especially in the distolingual area. The buccolingual dimension of the second molar is about the same, but mesiodistally it is noticeably narrower. It is also shorter occlusogingivally. The roots, however, are as long as those of the first molar. Its grinding function supplements that of the other molars.

2. Development Table: (Maxillary Second Molar)*

Initiation of calcification .... 2 1/2 to 3 years

Completion of enamel .... 7 to 8 years

Eruption .... 12 to 13 years

Completion of root .... 14 to 16 years

This tooth so closely resembles the first molar, only differences will be described.

3. Buccal aspect:

a. The crown is narrower both occlusogingivally and mesiodistally.

b. The buccal groove is located farther to the distal, resulting in a relatively larger mesiobuccal cusp, and a distobuccal cusp which is relatively sharper, but is smaller both in size and height.

c. Due to the diminished size of the distobuccal cusp, portions of the distal marginal ridge and distolingual cusp may be visible from the buccal aspect on some specimens.

4. Lingual aspect:

a. The distolingual cusp is much smaller in all dimensions than in the first molar. This feature allows much of the distobuccal cusp to be seen from the lingual. Occasionally, the distolingual cusp is entirely missing.

b. There is no cusp of Carabelli.

c. The distolingual groove does not extend so far mesially or cervically, thus terminating at a point which is occlusal and distal to the center of the lingual surface. On occasional specimens, the groove does not even extend onto the lingual surface.

*From Wheeler, R.C.: *Dental Anatomy, Physiology and Occlusion* (5th ed.; Philadelphia: W.B. Saunders Company, 1974).

5. Mesial aspect:

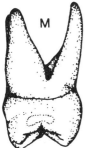

a. Occlusogingival crown length is less, but the buccolingual dimension is about the same as in the first molar.

b. The contact area is larger, because it is shared with a molar instead of a premolar. It is irregular, although somewhat ovoid, and wider buccolingually.

c. The cervical flattening or concavity seen on the first molar is never as pronounced, and is most often absent.

6. Distal aspect:

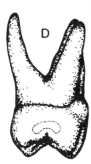

a. Due to the shorter and smaller distobuccal and distolingual cusps, more of the mesiobuccal and mesiolingual cusps is visible.

b. The cervical flattening or concavity is not normally present.

7. Occlusal aspect:

a. The crown is about the same width buccolingually, but is narrower mesiodistally which is at the expense of the distal structures.

b. There are two major types of crown form.

    i. <u>Rhomboidal</u> - The rhomboidal type looks much like the first molar, except the rhomboidal outline is more accentuated. This is the most common form.

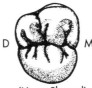

(Rhomboidal)

    ii. <u>Heart-shaped</u> - This type is similar to a typical third molar, with a very small distolingual cusp, and short distolingual groove. Sometimes the DL cusp is completely absent, and the distolingual groove is confined to the occlusal surface.

(Heart-Shaped)

c. Cusps, grooves, pits, etc. - With the exceptions previously noted, they are similar to, and named like those of the first molar. There are often more secondary grooves on the occlusal table of this tooth, however.

8. Roots:

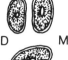

D   M

a. Root numbers and contours are similar to those of the first molar, and total root length may be equal to, or even greater, than in the first molar.

b. The two buccal roots are about the same length as each other, closer together, and more nearly parallel than in the first molar. They also exhibit more distal inclination, and there is a greater chance of their fusion.

c. The lingual root does not flare so much as in the first molar.

9. Variations and anomalies:

a. The heart-shaped occlusal form is the most common crown variation, and in this situation it is not unusual for the DL cusp to be absent.

b. Occasionally, a tubercle is found on the buccal surface.

c. The two buccal roots are sometimes fused together. Deflections and root curvatures are occasionally severe.

E. Permanent Maxillary Third Molar:

1. General characteristics:

a. Arch position - The upper third molar is located eighth and last from the midline in each maxillary quadrant of the permanent dentition. This tooth has a mesial contact with the permanent second molar, and no distal contact. It is not a succedaneous tooth.

b. Universal number:

Maxillary right third molar - #1

Maxillary left third molar - #16

c. General form and function - The crown of the third molar is generally smaller in all dimensions than the second molar, and it exhibits more rounding.

This is normally the smallest molar in the mouth, and the most variable tooth in the maxillary arch. The most common occlusal form is similar to the heart-shaped second molar.

The roots are normally shorter than those of the second molar, and are often partially, or fully fused.

Its function complements the other molars in grinding.

2. Development Table: (Maxillary Third Molar)*

Initiation of calcification .... 7 to 9 years

Completion of enamel .... 12 to 16 years

Eruption .... 17 to 21 years

Completion of root .... 18 to 25 years

3. Crown form:

a. When compared to the second molar, the crown is smaller in all dimensions, especially occlusocervically and mesiodistally.

b. This tooth varies so greatly that it is difficult to describe a standard, or typical third molar. Nevertheless, the heart-shaped form is the most common. The distolingual cusp is greatly diminished in size, or is absent, leaving only three functional cusps, and in many cases no distolingual groove. The groove pattern is variable, and often reveals many supplemental grooves.

---

*From Wheeler, R.C.: *Dental Anatomy, Physiology and Occlusion* (5th ed.; Philadelphia: W.B. Saunders Company, 1974).

c. Despite the variability in crown form, maxillary third molar specimens are almost always wider buccolingually than mesiodistally.

4. Root form:

a. Like crown form, root numbers and morphology are extremely variable. Root dimensions are normally the smallest of any maxillary molar.

b. The most common root type, usually in conjunction with the heart-shaped crown form, is three roots, which are often partially or wholly fused together.

5. Variations and Anomalies:

a. This tooth exhibits the most divergence in crown and root form of any maxillary tooth.

b. The crown varies in size from a simple, and tiny one cusp form, which is often devoid of grooves and pits, and is known as a peg third molar, to a large crown with numerous cusps, or tubercles, and an excessive number of randomly placed pits and grooves.

c. The number of root branches may vary from one, to as many as seven or eight. Root length and curvatures are also quite discrepant, and deflections at odd angles are common.

d. Third molars of both arches are often congenitally missing or impacted.

e. Supernumerary teeth - Although rare, supernumerary (extra) teeth are sometimes found just distal to the third molar area. When present, they are usually impacted.

Maxillary Right First Molar

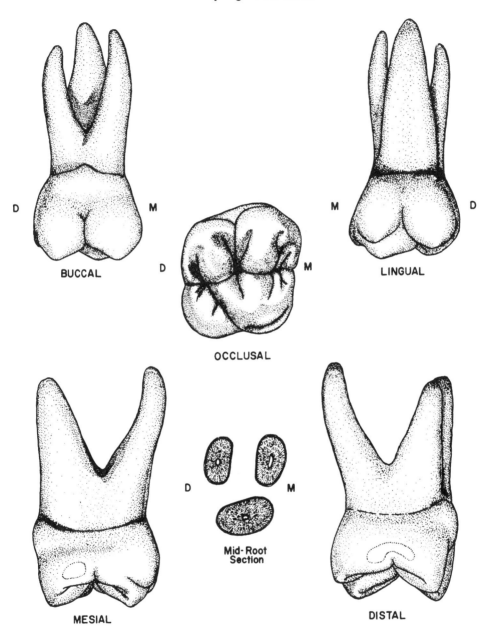

BUCCAL

D   M

D   M

OCCLUSAL

M   D

LINGUAL

MESIAL

D   M

Mid-Root Section

DISTAL

Maxillary Right Second Molar

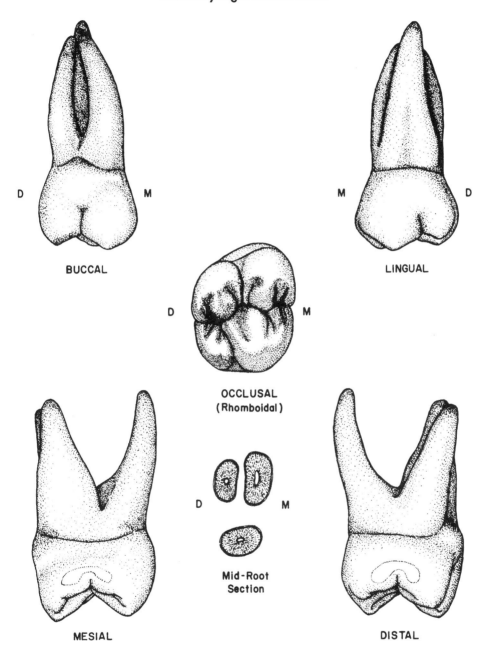

BUCCAL

LINGUAL

OCCLUSAL
(Rhomboidal)

MESIAL

Mid-Root
Section

DISTAL

113

Maxillary Right Third Molar
Three-Cusp Type

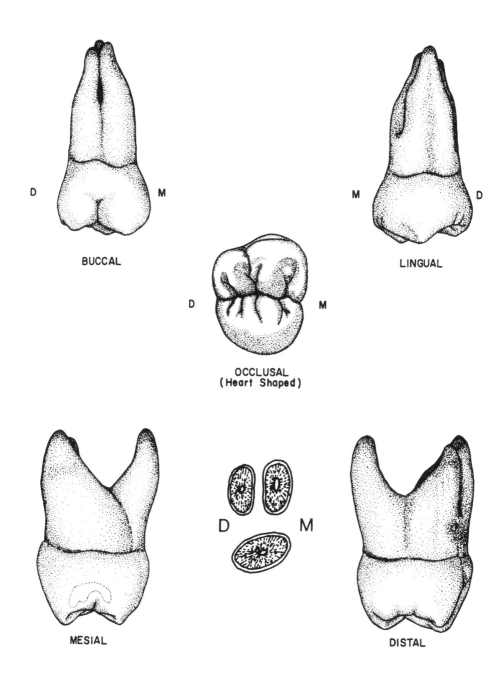

BUCCAL

LINGUAL

OCCLUSAL
(Heart Shaped)

MESIAL

DISTAL

Maxillary Right Third Molar
Four-Cusp Type

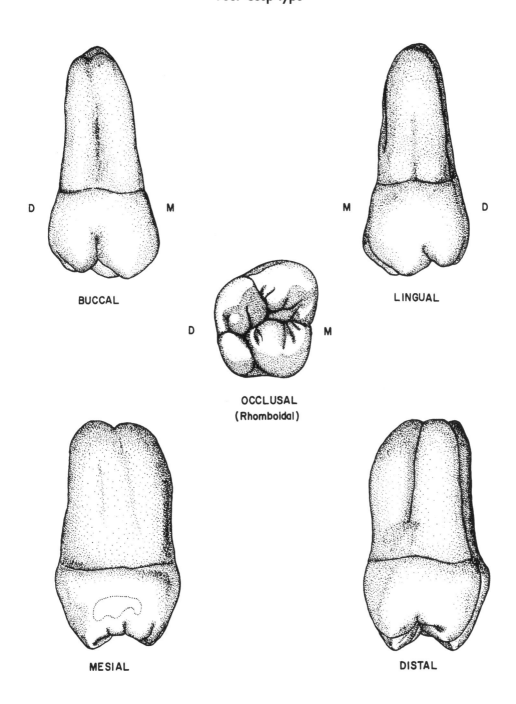

D BUCCAL M

M LINGUAL D

D OCCLUSAL M
(Rhomboidal)

MESIAL

DISTAL

Maxillary Right Third Molar
Continuous-Cusp Type

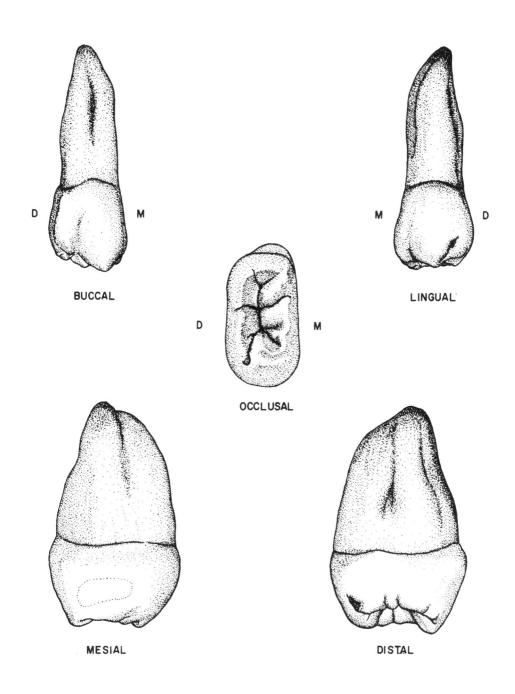

BUCCAL

D   M

OCCLUSAL

D   M

LINGUAL

M   D

MESIAL

DISTAL

UNIT # 8

I. **Reading Assignment:**

Unit # 8 (The Permanent Mandibular Molars)

II. **Specific Objectives:**

At the completion of this unit, the student will be able to:

A. List the appropriate age(s) concerning developmental chronology of the mandibular molars found in the development tables, or select the appropriate age(s) from a list, when given a certain developmental feature. The student should also be able to compare these ages among the mandibular molars.

B. Demonstrate a knowledge of the morphology of each surface of the crown, as well as the root, of each permanent mandibular molar by:

    1. describing,

    2. selecting the correct information from a list,

    3. or interpreting a diagram to identify or name any of the following features:

        a. Contours of any surface, or margin of any surface.

        b. Structural entities such as grooves, pits, ridges, inclined planes, cusps, fossae, lobes, etc.

        c. Height of contour and contact areas.

        d. Relative dimensions and shape.

        e. Any other surface feature.

        Furthermore, the student will be able to make comparisons of any of the above features between mandibular molars.

C. Make comparisons between permanent mandibular molars and other permanent teeth, where appropriate, by selecting the correct response from a list.

D. Make comparisons of the general characteristics of the mandibular molars, including function, arch position, distinguishing features, etc., by describing them, or selecting the correct response from a list, when given the tooth (teeth), or a description of the general characteristic(s).

E. Determine from a diagram or description whether a given permanent mandibular molar is first, second, or third, or right or left.

F. Determine the correct universal number or Palmer notation for a given diagram or description of any permanent mandibular molar.

G. Demonstrate a knowledge of any of the new terms in this unit, by defining them, or selecting the correct definition, or application thereof, from a list, when given the term, or any of its applications.

H. Demonstrate a knowledge of any of the variations or anomalies in this unit by describing them, or selecting the correct response from a list, when given the particular tooth (teeth), the anomaly, or any of its features or applications.

The student is also responsible for any material which was to have been mastered in previous units.

UNIT # 8
THE PERMANENT MANDIBULAR MOLARS

I.   **The Permanent Mandibular Molars:**

A.   Introduction:

1.   The permanent mandibular molars are the three most posterior teeth in each lower quadrant. Like their maxillary counterparts, they are named first (six-year) molar, second (twelve-year) molar, and third molar (wisdom tooth). They are the largest and strongest teeth in the mandibular arch. Mandibular molar crowns are much larger than those of mandibular premolars in all dimensions except occlusogingivally, where they are slightly shorter. Their general size normally decreases from first molar through third molar.

2.   The mandibular molars function with the maxillary molars in grinding, and their form, root structure, and bone support are suited to this role.

3.   A review of the features which serve to differentiate mandibular and maxillary molars includes:

a.   Crowns which are wider mesiodistally than buccolingually.

b.   Crowns which are rectangular or pentagonal from the occlusal aspect.

c.   Crowns which are rhomboidal and inclined to the lingual, from a proximal aspect.

d.   The presence of four or five major cusps, of which there are always two lingual cusps of approximately the same size.

e.   The presence of two roots in most cases.

B.   Permanent Mandibular First Molar:

1.   General characteristics:

a.   Arch position - The initial permanent tooth to erupt, the mandibular first molar is located sixth from the midline, and distal to the second deciduous molar. Hence it is not a succedaneous tooth. Because of its normal eruption time, it is often called a "six year" molar. The first molars are also thought of as the cornerstones of occlusion in the mandibular arch.

It shares a mesial contact with the deciduous second molar for approximately five years, until that tooth is replaced by the second premolar. There is no distal contact, until eruption of the permanent second molar occurs at about age twelve.

b.   Universal number:

Mandibular right first molar - #30

Mandibular left first molar - #19

c.   General form and function - The first molar is the largest and strongest tooth in the lower arch. It normally exhibits five functional cusps, and two well developed roots.

The crown is wider mesiodistally than buccolingually, and, in fact, the mesiodistal dimension is greater than that of any tooth in the mouth. The crown is relatively short occlusocervically, the only dimension which is normally less than that of the teeth anterior to it. It displays a trapezoidal outline from the buccal and lingual, and exhibits a rhomboidal form from either proximal aspect. From the occlusal, the general outline is pentagonal.

In mastication, it functions with the other molars in grinding.

2. Development Table: (Mandibular First Molar)*

Initiation of calcification .... at birth

Completion of enamel .... 2 1/2 to 3 years

Eruption .... 6 to 7 years

Completion of root .... 9 to 10 years

3. Buccal aspect:

a. General considerations - The buccal is the largest lateral surface of not only the mandibular first molar, but of any tooth in the mouth. It is trapezoidal in outline, with the greatest mesiodistal width at the occlusal. At least portions of all five cusps are visible from this aspect.

b. Mesial outline - The mesial outline is slightly concave from the contact area cervically, and convex occlusal to the contact. The height of contour of the mesial outline is located at the junction of the occlusal and middle thirds.

c. Distal outline - The distal margin is generally more convex than the mesial outline. In the occlusal portion, it is more rounded, and cervical to the contact area it is straight to slightly convex, as compared to the concavity of the mesial margin. The height of contour is found at a slightly more cervical location than that of the mesial margin, but it is still at the junction of the occlusal and middle thirds.

d. Cervical outline - The cervical line exhibits slight, but regular curvature apically, and sometimes displays a sharply pointed projection over the bifurcation area.

e. Occlusal outline - The occlusal margin is wider than the outline at the cervical. It is divided into three portions by two grooves, as they pass onto the buccal surface. They are termed buccal (mesiobuccal) groove, and distobuccal groove. The mesio-occlusal and disto-occlusal slopes of three cusps are present in the occlusal outline. The mesiobuccal and distobuccal cusp tips are relatively blunt, while the distal cusp is normally lower, and somewhat sharper than the other two.

f. Other considerations - The buccal surface itself is divided into three portions by the two grooves, and these three sections decrease in size posteriorly. The convex buccal cusp ridges of the three cusps are the most prominent features of the occlusal portion of each section, and they are separated by the occlusocervical concavities containing the two grooves.

Buccal (mesiobuccal) groove - This groove is located in a concavity between the convex buccal cusp ridges of the mesiobuccal and distobuccal cusps. From the occlusal outline, it extends straight cervically to a point about midway between the gingival and occlusal margins, but a little to the mesial of center in the mesiodistal dimension. It most often terminates in a buccal pit, but may fade out, or bifurcate into two angular grooves which themselves fade out after a short distance. The groove, as well as the pit, are sometimes deep and fissured.

Distobuccal groove - This groove is located in a concavity between the buccal ridge convexities of the distobuccal and distal cusps. It crosses the occlusal outline close to the distal margin, and then extends cervically and

D   M

---

*From Wheeler, R.C.: *Dental Anatomy, Physiology and Occlusion* (5th ed.; Philadelphia: W.B. Saunders Company, 1974).

119

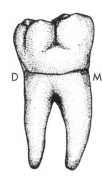

slightly distally to terminate at a point in the middle third near the distobuccal line angle. It normally ends in a distobuccal pit, but sometimes simply fades out.

Buccogingival ridge - As in the maxillary arch, this structure is not found on all first molar specimens. When present, it appears as a mesiodistal convexity in the cervical third of the buccal surface. It is usually more prominent in its mesial portion

Again, like the maxillary molars, there may be a shallow concavity which extends mesiodistally in the middle third. More specifically, it is located just occlusal to the buccogingival ridge in the area of termination of the two buccal grooves.

The height of contour is located in the cervical third.

4. Lingual aspect:

a. General considerations - The lingual surface is also roughly trapezoidal in outline, with the longer parallel side of the trapezoid at the occlusal. Since the crown is widest mesiodistally at the buccal, and its mesial and distal surfaces taper somewhat toward the lingual, portions of both proximal surfaces can be seen from this aspect. The lingual surface is, in fact, generally smaller than the buccal surface.

b. Mesial outline - The mesial outline is convex occlusal from the contact area, which is the crest of curvature, and is located at the junction of the occlusal and middle thirds. From the contact area cervically, it is concave.

c. Distal outline - The entire distal margin is convex, but especially so from the contact area occlusally, which is the outline of the distal portion of the distal cusp. The height of contour of the distal outline is also at the junction of the occlusal and middle thirds.

d. Cervical margin - The cervical line is shorter mesiodistally, and is located at a more occlusal level, than on the buccal surface. It is usually irregular and nearly straight, although it can display a pointed projection in the bifurcation area.

e. Occlusal margin - The occlusal outline is usually broken by the lingual groove passing onto the lingual surface. The mesiolingual and distolingual cusps, and a small portion of the distal cusp are visible from this aspect. The outline of the mesiolingual cusp is slightly wider than that of the distolingual cusp. The two lingual cusp tips are more pointed than the buccal cusp tips, and they are approximately equal in height.

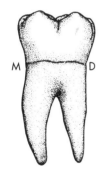

f. Other considerations - The lingual cusp ridges of the two lingual cusps are convex, with the shallow concavity containing the lingual groove lying between them in the occlusal third. Except for the concavity of the lingual groove, the occlusal and middle thirds of the surface are generally convex, but there is normally a flattened area in the center of the cervical third.

Lingual groove - This groove crosses from the occlusal surface onto the lingual surface slightly to the distal of center, extends cervically, and terminates in the occlusal third near its junction with the middle third. It usually fades out, but on rare occasions it ends in a lingual pit. Occasionally, the groove is confined to the occlusal surface and does not pass onto the lingual surface at all. It is shallower than either of the buccal grooves, and is seldom fissured on the lingual surface.

The lingual height of contour is located in the middle third.

5. Mesial aspect:

a. General considerations - Although the mesial surface is said to be rhomboidal, it is not a perfect rhomboid, since the surface is wider at the cervical than at the occlusal. From the mesial and distal aspects, the crown displays the lingual inclination which is unique to the mandibular posterior teeth. Only the two mesial cusps are visible from this aspect.

b. Buccal outline - The buccal margin is usually convex from gingival to occlusal, but is most convex at the cervical third crest of curvature, especially if the tooth has a buccocervical ridge. On some specimens there is a slight concavity in the middle third of the outline.

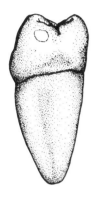

c. Lingual outline - The lingual outline is straight, or slightly convex, from the cervical margin to the height of contour in the middle third. It is quite convex occlusal to the height of contour.

d. Cervical margin - The CEJ may be either relatively straight, or slightly curved occlusally, but it is always located at a more occlusal level on the lingual side.

e. Occlusal margin - This margin is concave, and is composed of the mesial marginal ridge outline which is confluent with the mesial cusp ridges of the mesiobuccal and mesiolingual cusps. A mesial marginal groove is usually present.

f. Other considerations - A flattened, or slightly concave area, which is often triangular in form, is centrally located in the gingival third of the surface. It is not consistently as deep or as extensive as the mesial concavity of the maxillary first premolar.

The contact area is round to slightly ovoid in shape, and located slightly to the buccal at the middle and occlusal third junction.

The height of contour of the mesial surface is associated with the contact area at the junction of the occlusal and middle thirds.

6. Distal aspect:

a. General considerations - The distal surface is similar in outline to the mesial, and is also wider buccolingually at the cervical than at the occlusal. It is, however, generally smaller than the mesial surface, especially in the buccolingual dimension.

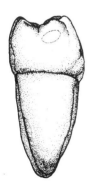

b. Buccal margin - The buccal margin is similar to that of the mesial aspect, except the concavity that is sometimes present in the middle third is not as evident when it is present.

c. Lingual outline - The lingual outline is comparable to that of the mesial aspect.

d. Cervical outline - The cervical line is relatively straight, although it may curve occlusally to a slight degree. As on the mesial surface, it is normally located at a more cervical level at its buccal extremity than at the lingual.

e. Occlusal outline - The occlusal outline is shorter than on the mesial, but similarly concave. The distal marginal ridge is notched by the distal marginal groove, which is shorter than the mesial marginal groove, and located to the lingual of center. The marginal ridge is sometimes difficult to separate from the outline of the distal cusp in the buccal portion of the occlusal outline. Therefore, the height of the distal marginal ridge is somewhat dependent on the prominence of the distal cusp. Normally, the ridge is located at a more cervical level than on the mesial, but the height is also more

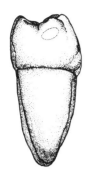

variable because of its relation to the distal cusp. The tip of the distal cusp is located toward the buccal, occlusal to the contact area.

f. Other considerations - Since the distal surface is shorter occluso-gingivally than the mesial, more of the occlusal surface may be seen. The distal cusp is the most prominent feature of this view, but portions of all five cusps are visible.

More of the buccal surface is likewise visible, since it converges toward the distal, resulting in a narrower buccolingual dimension. Because of the convergence of the buccal surface, the distobuccal groove is also visible from this aspect.

The distal contact area is located similarly to the mesial contact area. It is larger, since it contacts the second molar, as contrasted to the mesial contact with the second premolar. It is ovoid in outline, wider buccolingually than occlusocervically.

7. Occlusal aspect:

a. General considerations - The occlusal form is roughly pentagonal in shape. The distal portion of the buccal outline tapers toward the lingual, to create the fifth side of the outline. The crown is wider mesiodistally than buccolingually, and it is widest mesiodistally toward the buccal, and widest buccolingually toward the mesial.

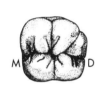

b. Buccal outline - The buccal outline is separated into three sections by the two buccal grooves. The relative length of the three portions decreases distally, so that the mesiobuccal is longest, distobuccal next, and the distal is shortest. The buccal line angles are quite rounded, especially when compared to those of anterior teeth and premolars.

c. Lingual outline - The lingual margin is divided into two slightly convex portions by the lingual groove. The mesial portion is slightly the longer of the two.

d. Mesial outline - The mesial outline is divided into two approximately equal segments by the mesial marginal groove.

e. Distal outline - The distal is the shortest of the four margins, and consists of two convexities, separated by the distal marginal groove.

f. Boundaries - The occlusal table is bounded proximally by the two marginal ridges, and on the buccal and lingual by the mesial and distal cusp ridges of the five cusps.

8. Components of the Occlusal Table:

a. Cusps - There are normally five cusps, all of which are functional, although the distal cusp is much smaller than the others. Despite its name, the distal cusp is grouped with the MB and DB cusps as one of the three "buccal" cusps. However, from the buccal or occlusal aspects, the reason for this grouping is evident.

i. Mesiobuccal cusp - The mesiobuccal is the bulkiest cusp, and the longest of the three buccal cusps, although rather blunt and rounded. The MB cusp has four cusp ridges which are described as follows:

Buccal cusp ridge - The buccal cusp ridge extends cervically from the cusp tip about halfway down the buccal surface.

Lingual cusp ridge - The lingual cusp ridge extends lingually to end at the mesial portion of the central groove. It is the longest and most prominent of the four ridges.

Mesial cusp ridge - This cusp ridge extends mesially to the mesio-bucco-occlusal point angle area.

Distal cusp ridge - It extends distally to the buccal groove.

ii. Distobuccal cusp - Except for the distal, the distobuccal cusp is the smallest of the cusps, and it has a rounded tip. The DB cusp has four cusp ridges which are described as follows:

Buccal cusp ridge - The buccal cusp ridge extends cervically from the cusp tip about halfway the width of the buccal surface.

Lingual cusp ridge - The lingual cusp ridge extends mesiolingually to the area of the central pit.

Mesial cusp ridge - This cusp ridge extends mesially to the buccal groove.

Distal cusp ridge - It extends distally to the distobuccal groove.

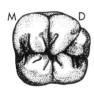

The four inclined planes of both the MB and DB cusps are named similarly to those of other posterior teeth. The inclined planes of the three buccal cusps are all functional, while only the buccal two are functional on the lingual cusps.

iii. Mesiolingual cusp - Along with the DL, the ML cusp is the longest and sharpest of the cusps, and it is second in size to the MB cusp. There are four cusp ridges which are described as follows:

Buccal cusp ridge - The buccal cusp ridge extends from the cusp tip distobuccally to end at the mesial portion of the central groove.

Lingual cusp ridge - The lingual cusp ridge extends cervically about halfway down the lingual surface.

Mesial cusp ridge - This cusp ridge extends mesially to the mesiolinguo-occlusal point angle area.

Distal cusp ridge - It extends distally to end at the lingual groove.

iv. Distolingual cusp - The DL cusp is quite sharp, but is slightly smaller in size than the mesiolingual cusp. The DL cusp has four cusp ridges, which are described as follows:

Buccal cusp ridge - The buccal cusp ridge extends from the cusp tip mesiobuccally to end in the area of the junction of the distobuccal groove and the distal portion of the central groove.

Lingual cusp ridge - It extends in a cervical direction to the middle third of the lingual surface.

Mesial cusp ridge - The mesial cusp ridge extends mesially to the lingual groove.

Distal cusp ridge - It extends distally to the distolinguo-occlusal point angle area.

v. Distal cusp - The distal cusp is much the smallest and shortest of the five cusps, but is relatively sharp. Its four cusp ridges are described as follows:

Buccal cusp ridge - The buccal cusp ridge runs in a cervical direction, and occupies much of the area surrounding the distobuccal line angle.

Lingual cusp ridge - It extends mesiolingually to end in the distal pit area. Compared to other triangular ridges of posterior teeth, it is short and poorly defined.

Mesial cusp ridge - The mesial cusp ridge extends from the cusp tip mesiobuccally to the distobuccal groove.

<u>Distal cusp ridge</u> - It forms the buccal portion of the distal border of the occlusal surface, and extends in a lingual direction rather than distally.

b. Cusp comparison:

i. Relative cusp length (height) from highest to lowest: The mesio-lingual and distolingual cusps are approximately the same height, followed by the mesiobuccal, distobuccal, and distal cusps.

ii. Relative cusp size (bulk) from largest to smallest: The mesiobuccal cusp is the largest cusp, followed in diminishing size by the mesiolingual, distolingual, distobuccal, and distal cusps.

c. Transverse ridges - There are no transverse ridges on the occlusal surface of the mandibular first molar.

d. Marginal ridges - The two marginal ridges are named <u>mesial</u> and <u>distal marginal ridges,</u> and enclose those limits of the occlusal surface.

e. Fossae - There are three recognizable fossae on the occlusal table, with the central fossa encompassing by far the largest area.

i. <u>Central fossa</u> - As the name implies, this fossa is located in the central portion of the occlusal table. It is somewhat circular in shape, and the largest and deepest of the three fossae. It is bounded by the triangular ridges of the four major cusps, as well as the distal cusp ridges of the MB and the ML cusps and the mesial cusp ridges of the DB and DL cusps.

ii. <u>Mesial triangular fossa</u> - The mesial triangular fossa has a location and limits similar to the same fossa on other posterior teeth. It is deeper and more distinct than the distal triangular fossa. Its boundaries include the mesial marginal ridge, the triangular ridges of the two mesial cusps, and the mesial cusp ridges of the two mesial cusps.

iii. <u>Distal triangular fossa</u> - Again, this fossa has a location similar to its counterparts on other posterior teeth. It is the shallowest and least distinct of the three occlusal fossae on this tooth. It is bounded by portions of the distal cusp and distal marginal ridge, as well as the triangular ridges of the D and DL cusps.

f. Pits and grooves - The occlusal surface of the first molar has the most complex groove pattern of any of the mandibular molars.

i. <u>Central pit</u> - The central pit is located in the central fossa, and is the deepest pit on the occlusal surface. It is situated midway mesiodistally, and more than halfway from buccal to lingual. It is at the junction of three primary developmental grooves:

<u>Mesiobuccal (Buccal) groove</u> - This groove extends from the central pit buccally onto the buccal surface. In its most lingual portion, it is confluent with the mesial portion of the central groove.

<u>Distobuccal groove</u> - The distobuccal groove extends in a distobuccal direction from the central pit onto the buccal surface. In its most lingual area, it is confluent with the distal portion of the central groove.

<u>Lingual groove</u> - The lingual groove extends from the central pit lingually onto the lingual surface.

ii. Mesial pit - The mesial pit is situated halfway buccolingually in the deepest area of the mesial triangular fossa. It is not as deep as the central pit. This pit is the junction of four developmental grooves.

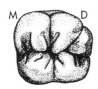

Central groove (Mesial portion) - The mesial portion of the central groove extends mesiobuccally from the central pit a short distance, via the mesiobuccal groove, and then after their separation, continues in a mesial direction to the mesial pit.

Mesiobuccal triangular groove - This groove is similar to the same groove as it was described for the maxillary molars.

Mesiolingual triangular groove - It is also similar to the same groove as it was described for the maxillary molars.

Mesial marginal groove - From the mesial pit, this groove crosses the mesial marginal ridge in a mesial direction.

iii. Distal Pit - The distal pit is located midway buccolingually in the depth of the distal triangular fossa. It is not so deep as the central or mesial pits. It is the union of three developmental grooves:

Central groove (Distal portion) - From the distal pit, this groove passes mesiobuccally to become confluent with the distobuccal groove.

Distolingual triangular groove - This groove extends from the distal pit toward the distolingual line angle, where it fades out.

Distal marginal groove - It extends distally from the distal pit over the distal marginal ridge.

Note: The central groove in entirety extends from the mesial pit to the distal pit, and includes its mesial portion, its distal portion, and segments of the mesiobuccal and distobuccal grooves.

9. Roots:

a. The mandibular first molar has a root trunk which bifurcates to form mesial and distal roots (branches). Both roots are widest buccolingually, and both may have developmental depressions on the mesial and distal root surfaces, termed longitudinal grooves, or root concavities. The two root branches are usually about the same length, but if one root is slightly longer, it invariably is the mesial root which is favored.

Normally, the two roots have some distal angulation, although occasionally they are nearly straight from the root trunk apically.

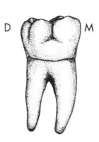

i. Mesial root - The mesial branch is the widest and strongest of the two roots. It curves mesially from the cervical line to the middle third, and then angles slightly distally to the apex. Its buccal and lingual surfaces are convex throughout their length, while the mesial and distal surfaces are flattened to concave, depending on the presence and prominence of longitudinal grooves.

ii. Distal root - The distal branch is generally smaller and weaker than the mesial root. It is usually straight, but on occasion it curves mesially or distally in the apical third. Normally, only the mesial root surface has a longitudinal groove. The buccal and lingual surfaces are convex throughout their length.

b. Mid root section - In cross section at this level, both roots are wider buccolingually, and the mesial root has a larger outline. The outline is convex buccally and lingually on both roots. Mesially and distally, the outline is flattened or concave, depending on the presence and prominence of longitudinal grooves.

10. Variations and Anomalies:

a. The first molar exhibits few developmental anomalies. However, on rare occasions, the crown may lack a distal cusp.

b. Mulberry molar - The mulberry molar, along with Hutchinson's incisor, are a consequence of congenital syphilis. On the first molars, the cusps are more centrally positioned on the occlusal table, creating a gnarled appearance.

c. Occasionally, the first molar exhibits three roots, when the mesial root has buccal and lingual branches.

C. Permanent Mandibular Second Molar:

1. General characteristics:

a. Arch position - The second molar is the seventh tooth from the midline in each mandibular quadrant. The mesial contact is shared with the permanent mandibular first molar, while distal contact with the permanent third molar occurs if and when that tooth erupts. It is also known as the "twelve year" molar, due to its normal time of eruption.

b. Universal number:

Mandibular right second molar - #31

Mandibular left second molar - #18

c. General form and function - The second molar resembles the first molar in many respects, although it is more symmetrical, and smaller in all dimensions. It has the least complicated occlusal design of any molar. Normally only four cusps are present, and thus there is no distobuccal groove, and no distal cusp.

The second molar complements the other molars in their grinding function.

2. Development Table: (Mandibular Second Molar)*

Initiation of calcification .... 2 1/2 to 3 years

Completion of enamel .... 7 to 8 years

Eruption .... 11 to 13 years

Completion of root .... 14 to 15 years

The second molar is so similar to the first molar that mostly contrasts with that tooth will be made.

3. Buccal aspect:

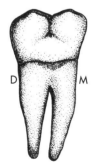

a. General considerations - The buccal surface is trapezoidal like that of the first molar, but is shorter occlusogingivally, and narrower mesiodistally.

b. Mesial margin - The mesial margin is similar to the first molar's. It is convex in the occlusal portion, and concave in the cervical portion.

c. Distal margin - Again, this outline is similar to that of the first molar. It is generally convex, and more so than the mesial margin.

d. Cervical margin - The cervical line normally has little curvature like that of the first molar, but some specimens may exhibit a sharp dip over the bifurcation area.

---

*From Wheeler, R.C.: *Dental Anatomy, Physiology and Occlusion* (5th ed.; Philadelphia: W.B. Saunders Company, 1974).

126

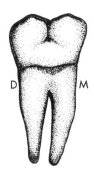

e. Occlusal margin - This margin is separated into two nearly equal halves by the buccal groove. The two buccal cusps, the mesiobuccal and distobuccal cusps, are about equal in length as are their cusp outlines.

f. Other considerations - The buccal groove breaks the occlusal outline at about its mesiodistal midpoint. It extends cervically to the middle third, where it normally terminates in a buccal pit, but may just fade out. There is no distobuccal groove.

The buccal cusp ridges of the two buccal cusps form occlusocervical convexities on either side of the concave area which contains the buccal groove.

When present, the buccogingival ridge is similar to that of the first molar, and is most prominent in its mesial portion.

There is normally no mesiodistal concavity in the middle third like some first molars exhibit, but some specimens do show a little flattening in this area.

The height of contour is located in the cervical third.

4. Lingual aspect:

a. General considerations - The lingual surface is also trapezoidal in outline. It is also shorter occlusocervically, and narrower mesiodistally than the first molar.

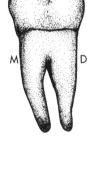

b. Mesial, distal, and cervical outlines are similar to those of the lingual surface of the first molar.

c. Occlusal outline - The occlusal outline is divided approximately in half by the lingual groove. Only the two lingual cusps are visible.

d. Other considerations - The lingual groove crosses the occlusal outline onto the lingual surface, and fades out in the occlusal third near its junction with the middle third.

Since the mesial and distal surfaces of the second molar crown converge only slightly toward the lingual, little, if any, of these surfaces is visible from the lingual aspect.

The height of contour in the middle third and other surface contours are similar to those of the first molar. There is often a centrally located concavity in the cervical third, which corresponds to the flattened area of the first molar.

5. Mesial aspect:

The mesial aspect is similar to the first molar except:

a. It is smaller in general size and is more convex in all directions.

b. The cervical outline is straighter, but like the first molar is more cervically positioned on the buccal as compared to the lingual.

c. The mesial contact area is definitely ovoid, when compared to the first molar's round or slightly ovoid mesial contact.

6. Distal aspect:

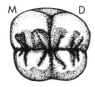

The distal aspect is comparable to the first molar except:

   a. There is no distal cusp contour, and no distobuccal groove.

   b. Since there is no distal cusp, the buccal surface shows much less convergence toward the distal. Consequently, the distal surface is about the same size as the mesial surface, and only a little of the cervical third of the buccal surface is visible.

   c. The contact area is centered on the surface both buccolingually and occlusogingivally. It is wider buccolingually than occlusocervically, but is more irregular in its configuration.

7. Occlusal aspect:

   a. General considerations - The occlusal table of most second molars is rectangular in shape, but the distal outline is more rounded, when compared to the slightly rounded mesial half. Even though the occlusal table itself is rectangular, the tooth outline from this aspect bulges at the mesiobuccal. This is due to the greater prominence of the mesial portion of the cervical height of contour, which is visible because of the lingual inclination of the crowns of mandibular posterior teeth. The design of the occlusal table and its anatomy are the simplest of any first or second molar.

   b. Buccal outline - The buccal outline exhibits a single convexity, which is usually greater toward the mesial.

   c. Lingual margin - The lingual outline is slightly shorter than the buccal, and is divided into two equal segments by the lingual groove.

   d. Mesial margin - Mesially, the outline presents two portions, separated by the mesial marginal groove.

   e. Distal margin - The distal is slightly shorter than the mesial margin, and displays more convexity.

   f. Boundaries - The occlusal table is bounded by the two marginal ridges, along with the mesial and distal cusp ridges of all four cusps.

8. Components of the occlusal table:

   a. Cusps - There are normally four cusps on the mandibular second molar, all of which are functional.

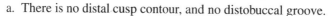

   i. The cusps are termed <u>mesiobuccal, distobuccal, mesiolingual</u>, and <u>distolingual</u>, and are fairly symmetrical in their position on the occlusal surface.

   ii. They are more nearly equal in size than the cusps of the first molar. Even so, the mesiobuccal cusp is normally the largest, while the distolingual cusp is normally the smallest, but its size may vary the most.

   iii. The buccal cusp ridges of the buccal cusps and the lingual cusp ridges of the lingual cusps are similar to the cusp ridges of the same four cusps on the first molar. The lingual cusp ridges of the buccal cusps meet the buccal cusp ridges of the lingual cusps to form two transverse ridges. Inclined planes, and whether they are functional or not, compare directly with the first molar. The mesial and distal cusp ridges of all cusps either meet each other (example: the mesial cusp ridge of the distobuccal cusp meets the distal cusp ridge of the mesiobuccal cusp in the buccal groove area), or they extend to the point angles (example: The mesial cusp ridge of the mesiobuccal cusp extends to the mesiobucco-occlusal point angle).

b. Marginal ridges - There are two marginal ridges which are similar to, and named the same, as those of other posterior teeth.

c. Transverse ridges - The two transverse ridges are formed by the union of the lingual cusp ridges of the buccal cusps and the buccal cusp ridges of the lingual cusps in the central groove area.

d. Fossae - The three fossae are named and located similar to those of the first molar, although the central fossa is more regular in shape.

e. Pits and grooves - Unlike the first molar, the major groove pattern is almost symmetrical, with the central groove and the buccal and lingual grooves combining to form a cross pattern, the intersection of which is in the central pit. There are often more supplemental grooves on the second molar, however.

    i. <u>Central pit</u> - The central pit is aptly named, because it is located centrally on the occlusal surface. It is the deepest of the three pits, and is formed by the junction of three developmental grooves:

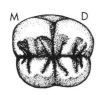

<u>Buccal groove</u> - The buccal groove extends buccally from the central pit onto the buccal surface.

<u>Lingual groove</u> - The lingual groove extends lingually from the central pit onto the lingual surface.

<u>Central groove</u> - It extends between the mesial and distal pits in a straight line which passes through the central pit. The central groove has mesial and distal portions separated by the central pit.

    ii. <u>Mesial pit</u> - The mesial pit is not as deep as the central pit, and is located midway buccolingually in the depth of the mesial triangular fossa. It is formed by the junction of four developmental grooves:

<u>Central groove</u> (Mesial portion)

<u>Mesiobuccal triangular groove</u>

<u>Mesiolingual triangular groove</u>

<u>Mesial marginal groove</u>

These grooves are located similarly to those of other posterior teeth. This is also true of the grooves which form the distal pit.

    iii. <u>Distal pit</u> - The distal pit resembles the mesial pit in depth and relative location, and is the junction of four developmental grooves:

<u>Central groove</u> (Distal portion)

<u>Distobuccal triangular groove</u>

<u>Distolingual triangular groove</u>

<u>Distal marginal groove</u>

9.   Roots:

The root structure of the second molar is similar to that of the first molar, with the following exceptions:

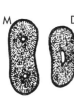

a. Usually the roots are shorter, but there is more variation, and they can occasionally even be longer.

b. The two branches are closer together, and thus their partial or total fusion is more common.

c. They usually have a greater distal angulation than the roots of the first molar.

129

10. Variations and Anomalies:

a. Crown anomalies are uncommon, although five-cusp specimens are occasionally seen.

b. Root anomalies are more common, and may be manifested in fused roots or irregular curvatures.

D. Permanent Mandibular Third Molar:

1. General characteristics:

a. Arch position - The mandibular third molar occupies the eighth, and last, position from the midline in each mandibular quadrant. The mesial contact area is shared with the permanent second molar, and there is no distal contact. It is also known as the lower "wisdom tooth."

b. Universal number:

Mandibular right third molar - #32

Mandibular left third molar - #17

c. General form and function - The mandibular third molars are extremely variable in size and shape of both their crown and root. However, they have one feature which remains constant in the midst of all the variation. Almost always, the mesiodistal dimension of the crown is greater than the bucco–lingual dimension, just the opposite of the maxillary third molar's dimensions.

Ordinarily, the molars decrease in general size from first molar to third molar, but the crowns of third molars can range from very small to much larger than any other molar. When third molars do vary greatly from normal size, it is more common to find extra large mandibular third molars, and extra small maxillary third molars.

2. Development Table: (Mandibular Third Molar)*

Initiation of calcification .... 8 to 10 years

Completion of enamel .... 12 to 16 years

Eruption .... 17 to 21 years

Completion of root .... 18 to 25 years

3. Crown form - The crown form is so variable that only generalizations about two basic types will be made.

a. Type I - The type I crown resembles the permanent second molar. It has four cusps, and the same general contours and occlusal pattern.

b. Type II - This type resembles the permanent first molar with five cusps, a similar occlusal pattern, and comparable contours.

c. Third molars normally exhibit many more secondary grooves on the occlusal table, and it is even sometimes difficult to identify the primary grooves.

d. The most common third molar reveals a Type I crown in conjunction with two root branches. Other crown forms range from one-cusped dwarfs to six-cusped specimens.

4. Roots:

a. Roots are also extremely variable in numbers, size, and curvatures. Single fused roots are common, as are two-rooted specimens similar to other man-

---

*From Wheeler, R.C.: *Dental Anatomy, Physiology and Occlusion* (5th ed.; Philadelphia: W.B. Saunders Company, 1974).

dibular molars. There may be as many as eight roots, and curvatures and fusions, or partial fusions, run the gamut.

b. Most often, root length is less than with other mandibular molars, regardless of the crown size. The most common root form reveals two short root branches.

5. Variations and Anomalies:

a. Third molars are often <u>congenitally missing</u> or <u>impacted</u>.

b. The area immediately distal to the third molar may be the site of <u>supernumerary teeth</u>. When present, they are normally impacted.

c. Many of the numerous anomalies have been mentioned previously, but almost any structural anomaly conceivable is possible in third molars.

Mandibular Right First Molar

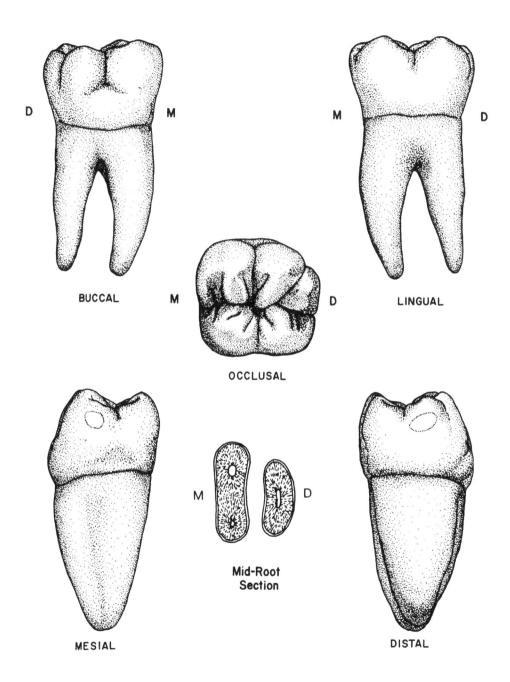

BUCCAL

M OCCLUSAL D

LINGUAL

MESIAL

Mid-Root
Section

DISTAL

Mandibular Right Second Molar

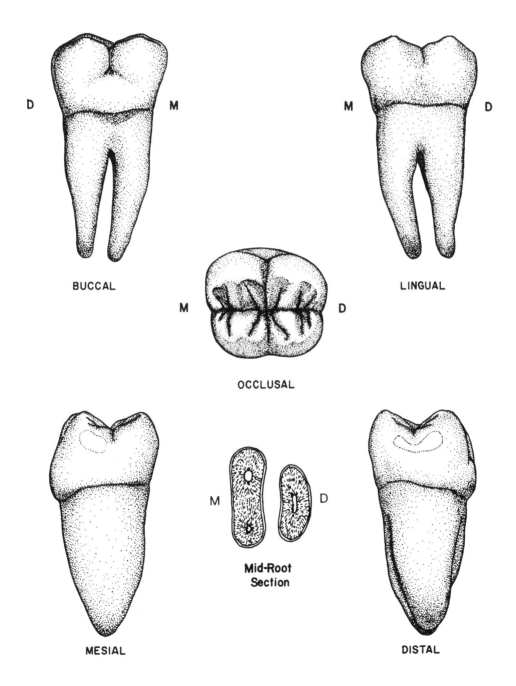

BUCCAL

LINGUAL

OCCLUSAL

MESIAL

Mid-Root
Section

DISTAL

TYPE I
Mandibular Right Third Molar
Four-Cusp type
with Fused Root

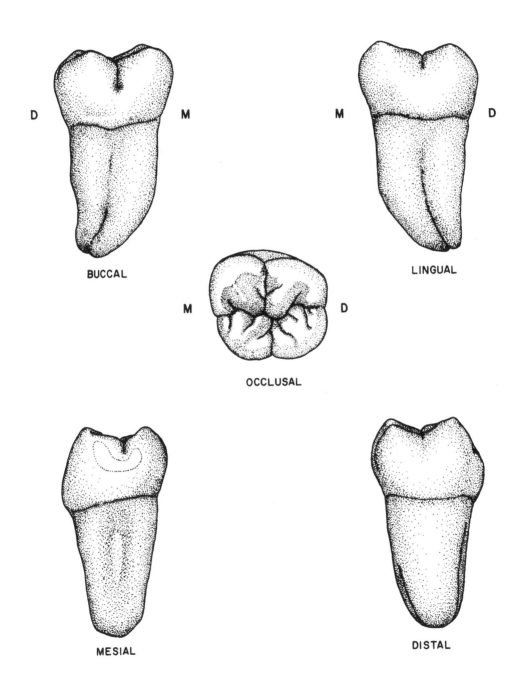

BUCCAL

LINGUAL

OCCLUSAL

MESIAL

DISTAL

TYPE II
Mandibular Right Third Molar
Five-Cusp Type
with Two Roots

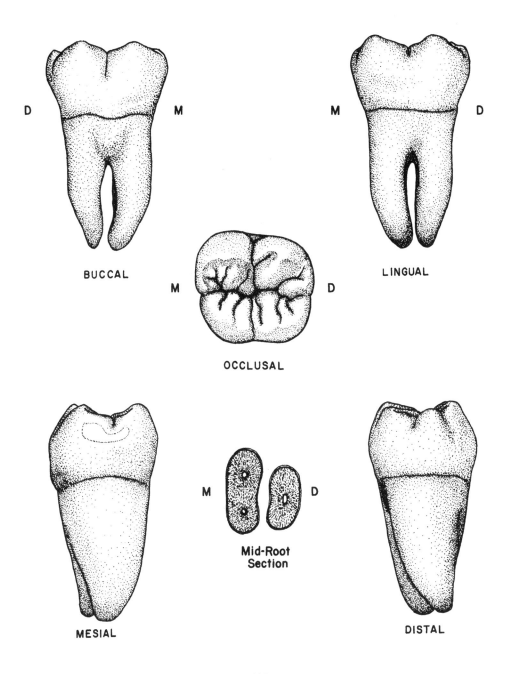

BUCCAL

LINGUAL

OCCLUSAL

MESIAL

Mid-Root
Section

DISTAL

UNIT # 9

I. **Reading Assignment:**

Unit # 9 (Pulp Cavities)

II. **Specific Objectives:**

At the completion of this unit, the student will be able to:

A. Define any of the anatomical terms relating to the pulp, or select the correct definition, or application thereof, from a list, when given the term or a description or application of a term.

B. List the main functions of the pulp, or differentiate between them by selecting the correct response from a list, when given the function or any of its applications.

C. Describe, or choose the correct response from a list concerning the changes which occur in the pulp and pulp cavity due to development, aging, or pathology.

D. Differentiate between the various pulp sections by describing or selecting the correct response from a list regarding their feasibility by x-ray, or any of their advantages or disadvantages.

E. Identify from a diagram or written description of any of the common sections of the pulp cavity, which permanent tooth is being described or diagrammed.

F. Demonstrate a knowledge of the normal pulpal anatomy and morphology for all the individual permanent teeth by describing it, selecting the correct response from a list, or making comparisons among the permanent teeth, when given a description of the anatomical feature. Anatomy and morphology include numbers, locations, shapes, outlines, relative thickness and lengths of pulp cavities, pulp horns, pulp chambers, chamber floors, orifices, pulp canals, and apical foramina, in any of the common sections or views.

G. Demonstrate a knowledge of the commonly observed differences from normal pulpal morphology for any of the individual permanent teeth by describing them for any tooth or group of teeth, or by selecting the correct response from a list, when given the normal anatomy or the deviations from normal.

H. Demonstrate a knowledge of the anatomy and components of a normal maxillary molar triangle by identifying them from a diagram or description.

The student is also responsible for any material which was to have been mastered in previous units.

UNIT # 9
PULP CAVITIES

I.   **Introduction:**

"Not all can be seen by observing the surface" is a statement that is sometimes equated to icebergs, but is likewise applicable to teeth, since only their surface features are evident to clinical inspection. A large segment of dental practice, namely <u>endodontia</u>, is directly concerned with the "hidden" portion of a tooth. The name, endodontia, implies "inside a tooth", thereby involving the treatment of the pulp cavity and its tissues.

As a prerequisite to the study of endodontic technique, it is imperative that the clinician is familiar with the anatomy and morphology of the pulp cavities of teeth. To properly perform root canal therapy, the clinician must possess accurate knowledge of not only the normal number of root canals, but also normal dimensions, contours, and shapes of the pulp cavities of the entire permanent dentition. Knowledge of the common variations and anomalies of pulp cavity anatomy is likewise essential. To point up the critical need for a working knowledge of pulp cavity morphology, endodontic failures are most often ascribed to improperly instrumented canals, and to undiscovered, and thus uninstrumented, supplementary canals.

This background becomes even more important when it is realized that endodontia involves an area in which direct vision is not possible. The radiograph (x-ray) is extremely useful, but has certain technical limitations. A major drawback focuses on the fact that routine x-rays can only outline pulp cavities in a mesiodistal cross section. In addition, superimposed structures may interfere with the interpretation of pulpal detail.

The relationship of the pulp cavity to endodontia has been emphasized, but it should be pointed out that most of this same knowledge is also necessary to competently practice in other areas of dentistry. For example, in restorative dentistry the clinician must constantly be aware of the location of the pulp when planning and performing treatment.

Therefore, the general objective of this unit is to prepare the student for advanced study in the dental curriculum by providing the necessary background about normal pulpal morphology and some of the common variations.

II.   **The Pulp Tissue and Pulp Cavity:**

A.   Introduction:

It is not the purpose of this section to preempt the basic sciences by describing pulp histology and physiology in detail. Hence, only a very brief review of the salient features will be presented.

B.   Anatomy of the Pulp Cavity:

The <u>pulp tissue</u> is the soft connective tissue which is found in the central portion of the tooth, entirely surrounded by dentin. The cavity, or space, in which the pulp tissue is located is divided into the following anatomical entities.

   1.   <u>Pulp cavity</u> - The pulp cavity is the entire central space in the dentin of a tooth, both root and crown, which contains the pulp tissue in a vital tooth. The outline of the pulp cavity generally corresponds to the external contour of the tooth, especially in newly erupted teeth. However, its size and contour in any individual tooth is related to the extent that normal physiologic aging has occurred, and that external factors such as pathology and occlusion have stimulated secondary dentin production.

   2.   <u>Pulp chamber</u> - The portion of the pulp cavity which is located roughly in

the anatomical crown of the tooth. It is normally larger in diameter than any portions of the pulp cavity found in roots.

3.   Pulp canal(s) - The section of the pulp cavity which is located basically in the anatomical root of the tooth, or in other words, that portion which is apical to the pulp chamber. Another term which is appropriate is root canal.

4.   Pulp horn(s) - The pulp horns are the pointed incisal (occlusal) limits of the pulp cavity and pulp chamber, which actually look like horns in many cases. They often reflect the lobe and cusp pattern of a tooth's crown.

5.   Apical foramen (pl.-foramina) - The constricted opening(s), at, or near the root apex, through which the main nutrient and nervous supply to the pulp enter and exit. The apical foramen is thus the apical limit of the pulp cavity.

6.   Lateral (Accessory) canals - Minute canals which usually extend in a lateral or roughly horizontal direction from the pulp to the periodontal membrane. They are most often found in the apical half of the root, and are a minor source of nutrient supply to the pulp.

7.   Supplementary canal - A root canal, or branch, which is in excess of the normal number of root canals found in a root. They serve the same functions as the main root canal(s), but are not present in all teeth.

8.   Anastomosis (pl.-anastomoses) - An extra canal branch which horizontally connects pulp canals with each other, or with supplementary canals.

C.   Physiology of the Pulp Tissue:

The pulp tissue functions in four major capacities for the dental organ:

1.   Formation of dentin: The dentinogenesis process is a function of the odontoblasts, which are cells that differentiate from the peripheral portion of the pulp. The primary dentin is normally laid down only during the period of tooth formation and ends when root development is complete. All dentin production does not necessarily cease following tooth maturation, however. The pulp is still capable of initiating the formation of secondary dentin at any time during the rest of its life, in both primary and permanent teeth. There are two types of secondary dentin, reparative and physiological, which differ from each other histologically, and from primary dentin both macroscopically (mainly color) and microscopically. Reparative dentin forms in response to acute or chronic irritants such as caries, thermal and functional trauma, and mechanical causes. In reality, this is a defensive and protective mechanism. Physiological secondary dentin may be deposited in a rather consistent and uniform manner, as a normal phenomenon of the aging process.

2.   Nutrition - This function maintains pulpal vitality, and is carried on by the blood and lymph vessels found in the pulp tissue. Their entrance and exit to the pulp cavity is chiefly through the apical foramen. There is some auxillary supply from the periodontal membrane.

3.   Sensation - The nerve tissue found in the pulp is responsible for relaying sensations to the brain centers. Not only do pain sensations occur, but the sensory function of the entire masticatory mechanism is coordinated.

4.   Defense and Protection - The pulp is capable of responding to an irritant, such as progressive caries, through inflammation, which is the classic defense mechanism of the body. This process may eventually result in the differentiation of odontoblasts, and the formation of reparative secondary dentin.

D.   Pulp Canal Development:

Early in the development of the root, the pulp canal is funnel-shaped at the root apex, with the greatest width of the funnel at the apex. Consequently, during much of the period of root development the pulp canal is widest in diameter at the apex. For this reason, endodontic therapy is difficult to perform successfully during this period, and is normally postponed until root formation has ceased. The completion of the apical portion of the root continues with primary dentin deposition, and the funnel-shaped opening is filled in until only a small opening, the apical foramen, is present. This is the point in time when root and root canal development are considered to be complete.

E.   Changes in the pulp cavity with age:

As previously indicated, the pulp tissue maintains the capacity to produce dentin as long as the pulp remains vital. This is secondary dentin, as contrasted to the primary dentin produced during tooth development. Secondary dentin production reduces the dimensions of the pulp cavity, which may be either in the form of a general reduction in size (physiological), or specific to an area of stimulation (reparative). When one, or both of these processes is occurring, pulp cavity dimensions are reduced. In the young tooth, the pulp horns are prominent elongations of the pulp chamber. With age, these extensions are often blunted, and sometimes even obliterated, so that the teeth of older individuals may not exhibit pulp horns. The same is true of the remainder of the pulp cavity, so that as the tooth ages, the pulp cavity normally decreases in size.

III.   **Sectioning of the Pulp Cavity:**

In the remaining text of this unit, pulp cavity anatomy will be described for individual permanent teeth. It is necessary, then, to briefly discuss the various views of the pulp cavity which may be produced by sections through different areas of the tooth.

As was previously mentioned, normal periapical radiographs (x-rays) of the teeth are taken in a faciolingual direction, thus outlining the pulp cavity in a mesiodistal section. However, the pulpal contours from this aspect are less variable than are those from a proximal aspect. Consequently, faciolingual sections exhibit more variability. Unfortunately, faciolingual sections are not normally feasible to the practitioner through x-rays.

Besides the mesiodistal and faciolingual sections which are vertical, knowledge of the anatomy in horizontal cross sections, at various levels of the pulp cavity, is valuable. Again, these cross sections are not possible with ordinary x-ray techniques. During the next section of the text, cross sections through the cervical line area and mid root level will be described for each tooth. These cross sections would be a welcome addition to the armamentarium of the endodontist, especially the mid-root section, which would most likely reveal the presence of supplementary root canals.

IV.   **Pulp Cavities of the Individual Permanent Teeth:**

A.   Introduction:

1.   The outline of the pulp cavity generally corresponds to the external contour of the tooth. This is very important, since it provides some knowledge of the contour of the pulp cavity without direct vision of it. In addition, the necessary background should be fresh in the student's mind with completion of the immediately preceding units on individual permanent teeth. The general shape of the crown can be utilized to provide a good indication of the shape and dimensions of the pulp chamber. For example, in anterior teeth where the labial and lingual surfaces are trapezoidal and widest at the incisal, the pulp chamber

is also widest toward the incisal. From either proximal, the pulp chamber is pointed at the incisal, and widest at the cervical, corresponding to the triangular-shaped proximal surfaces of anterior teeth. So, if the external anatomy of the teeth just studied is kept in mind, it will be easier to relate to the contours and dimensions of the pulp cavity. Cuspal anatomy can even be used to determine the heights and contours of the pulp horns, especially in posterior teeth.

2.   Another general rule suggests that in multirooted teeth there will be at least one root canal in each root branch. Furthermore, tooth roots with round cross sectional outlines generally possess one canal, whereas roots with oval or elongated cross sectional outlines often contain more than one canal.

B.   Maxillary Incisors:

   1.   Introduction:

Similarity between the pulp cavities of the maxillary central and lateral incisors is marked, since their general form is so similar. The pulp cavity outline reflects the external surface outline, as is generally the case with all teeth. The only real difference, excluding relative size, concerns pulp horn anatomy, where, the newly erupted central incisor normally exhibits three pulp horns, and the lateral incisor most often reveals either two or none. The pulp chamber is wider mesiodistally, in contrast to the maxillary canine and premolars, where the chamber is normally wider faciolingually.

   2.   Labiolingual Section:

   a. Pulp chamber - At its incisal extremity, the pulp chamber is pointed, and gradually thickens to its widest point at about the mid cingulum level. The labial outline is slightly convex, while on the lingual there is usually a rounded hump which corresponds to the external contour of the cingulum.

   b. Pulp canal - From approximately the cervical line, the outline of the single pulp canal tapers evenly to the apical foramen, generally following the contour of the root. The foramen is quite constricted, except in young teeth.

   3.   Mesiodistal Section:

   a. Pulp chamber - From this aspect, the chamber outline is widest at the incisal, and tapers fairly evenly to the cervical line level. The three pulp horns, corresponding to the three labial lobes, are prominent and pointed in young central incisors (laterals have two or none). In some specimens there is a slight mesiodistal widening, or bulge, at the cervical line. The mesiodistal dimension of the pulp chamber is generally greater than the labiolingual dimension.

   b. Pulp canal - From the cervical line, the pulp canal outline tapers rather evenly to the constricted apical foramen, again following the external root contour.

   4.   Cervical Cross Section - In newly erupted centrals, the pulp outline may be somewhat triangular like the root outline, but with age, the outline becomes generally circular. The outline for the lateral incisor is most often round at all ages.

   5.   Mid Root Cross Section - At this level, the pulp outline of both maxillary incisors is round.

C. Maxillary Canine:

1. Introduction:

The pulp cavity is similar in many respects to that of the maxillary incisors. The major difference reveals the pulp chamber width to be greater labiolingually than mesiodistally, the opposite of the incisors. In fact, the pulp cavity of the maxillary canine has the greatest faciolingual width of any anterior tooth. Since this tooth has the longest root in the mouth, it follows that its root canal is also longest.

2. Labiolingual Section:

a. Pulp chamber - The pulp outline is pointed incisally, and widens to the mid cingulum level, similar to the incisors. The labial margin is normally slightly convex, and there may be a slight bulging lingually in the cingulum area. The pointed incisal becomes rounded with age.

b. Pulp canal - Inasmuch as the root of this tooth is wider labiolingually than that of the incisors, the pulp canal is also wider in this dimension. At the apical third level, the canal becomes greatly constricted, although the foramen size is still larger than that of the incisors.

3. Mesiodistal Section:

a. Pulp chamber - In this section, the pulp cavity differs more from the incisors. From the pointed or slightly rounded incisal limit, the outline increases to its greatest width near the cervical line level. There are no pulp horns, as in the incisors, but the somewhat pointed incisal limit does correspond to the single cusp. Its narrowest dimension is at the incisal.

b. Pulp canal - From the cervical line to about the apical third level, the canal outline is about the same width, but in the apical third it tapers to the single foramen.

4. Cervical Cross Section - Since the root is ovoid and wider labiolingually, so is the pulp outline at this level.

5. Mid Root Cross Section - At this level, the pulp outline is less ovoid, and on occasion is nearly circular.

D. Maxillary First Premolar:

1. Introduction:

The maxillary first premolar has a pulp chamber which is considerably wider faciolingually than mesiodistally. This tooth is the only premolar which exhibits two roots in a majority of cases. Maybe this is why there is a wide variation in its pulp canal morphology. Recent research has revealed that about 70% of these teeth have two root canals with separate foramina, while less than 10% possess a single canal and foramen. It is interesting to note that nearly 5% display three canals, usually when there are three root branches. The remaining specimens exhibit two canals which unite in the apical third to exit a single foramen. One study also pointed out a large number of lateral canals, with about 50% of the cases displaying them. Because it is by far the most common situation, two fully formed canals will be described as representative of this tooth.

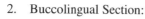

2. Buccolingual Section:

a. Pulp chamber - Occlusally, the chamber outline reveals two prominent pulp horns representing the two cusps and appropriately named buccal and lingual. The buccal horn is usually larger, and there is a concavity in outline between the two horns. From the pulp horn area, the chamber maintains a similar width to its <u>floor</u>, which is most often just apical to the cervical line.

b. Pulp canals - From the floor of the pulp chamber, the two root canals taper evenly to their apices. The lingual canal is usually slightly wider, even though the lingual root is most often smaller than the buccal root.

3. Mesiodistal Section:

a. Pulp chamber - The mesiodistal outline is quite similar to that of the maxillary canine, although it is shorter and slightly narrower.

b. Pulp canals - This outline is also similar to that of the canine. Only the buccal canal is visible from the buccal aspect, and likewise only the lingual canal can be seen in a section through the lingual part of the tooth.

4. Cervical Cross Section - The root outline at this level is wider buccolingually and is normally somewhat kidney shaped because of the tooth's mesial concavity, and the pulp outline follows that of the root. The maxillary first premolar exhibits two orifices in most cases, with the lingual orifice being slightly larger in size. <u>Orifice</u> is defined as the opening in the floor of the pulp chamber where a root canal exits.

5. Mid Root Cross Section - At this level, the two root outlines, and their respective canals, are both generally round, with the lingual canal normally slightly larger in diameter.

  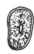

2-roots   Single

E. Maxillary Second Premolar:

1. Introduction:

The pulp cavity is again wider faciolingually than mesiodistally. The normal maxillary second premolar has but one root and one root canal, although often enough to be of significance the canal branches, usually in the apical third, and there are two foramina.

2. Buccolingual Section:

a. Pulp chamber - The outline is very similar to the first premolar's, and occlusally shows two pulp horns, of which the buccal horn is usually the larger.

b. Pulp canal - From the cervical line, the canal tapers regularly to the apical third, where it becomes constricted. The foramen is normally larger than either of the foramina of the first premolar. Occasionally, the canal branches, but rejoins in the apical third, and occasionally there is an apical third branching with two separate foramina. On rare occasions, there may be two roots, and two root canals, similar to the most common type of first premolar.

3. Mesiodistal Section - It is almost identical to the maxillary canine and first premolar from this aspect.

142

4. Cervical Cross Section - Since the single root is more ovoid, and not kidney shaped like the first premolar, the canal is also somewhat oval, but much wider buccolingually than mesiodistally.

5. Mid Root Cross Section - The normal outline reveals one canal which is ovoid, and wider buccolingually than mesiodistally.

F. Maxillary First Molar:

1. Introduction:

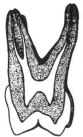

MESIAL VIEW

Since the crown of maxillary molars is generally wider buccolingually, it is not surprising that the pulp chamber is also wider in this dimension. Until recently, it was thought that the maxillary first molar seldom deviated from a situation of one root canal in each of its three roots. In the past few years, exacting research has disproved that belief. It has been shown that the MB root exhibits two root canals in about 60% of the specimens studied, and only one in the other 40%.

2. Buccolingual Section - The buccolingual section will be described from the mesial aspect for a cut taken through the MB and lingual roots. The distal aspect, with a section through the DB and lingual roots, is similar, except that only one canal is normally present in the DB root, and the DL pulp horn is much less prominent than the DB horn. The cusp of Carabelli is not normally represented by a pulp horn.

a. Pulp chamber - Mesiobuccal and mesiolingual pulp horns are visible from this aspect and they are nearly equal in height. The chamber outline tapers slightly from the cervical line floor toward the occlusal, so it is normally widest at the cervical, similar to the trapezoidal outline of the mesial crown surface.

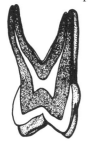

DISTAL VIEW

b. Pulp canals - In the majority (about 60%) of the specimens, two MB root canals are evident. Most often, the two MB canals will reunite in the apical third and exit via a common foramen. In about 40% of the maxillary first molars, only one MB canal will exist. Also visible in this section is the lingual root canal, which tapers evenly to its foramen. There is normally much greater flare between the buccal and lingual root canals in this view than there is between the MB and DB canals in a mesiodistal section.

3. Mesiodistal Section - Only the mesiodistal section from the buccal aspect will be considered. It should be pointed out that in the lingual view of a mesiodistal section, the only canal evident is the lingual canal, and its outline is generally wider than it is in a buccolingual section.

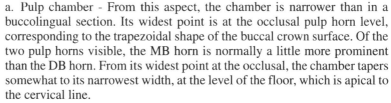

BUCCAL VIEW

a. Pulp chamber - From this aspect, the chamber is narrower than in a buccolingual section. Its widest point is at the occlusal pulp horn level, corresponding to the trapezoidal shape of the buccal crown surface. Of the two pulp horns visible, the MB horn is normally a little more prominent than the DB horn. From its widest point at the occlusal, the chamber tapers somewhat to its narrowest width, at the level of the floor, which is apical to the cervical line.

b. Pulp canals - Even if the MB root has two canals, normally only one of them is visible in this view. However, any buccal canals (MB and DB) are more constricted than the lingual canal, and they follow the external root curvatures to their restricted apices. When single, the MB canal is usually wider than the DB canal.

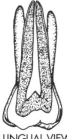

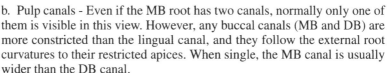

LINGUAL VIEW

143

4.   Cervical Line Cross Section - At the cervical line level, the outline of the pulp cavity is roughly rhomboidal in shape. However, the floor of the chamber is located in the root trunk at a more apical level than the cervical line, and exhibits three root canal <u>orifices</u>. Even when two MB canals are present, there is normally but a single MB orifice. These openings are arranged in a typical triangular shape, known as the <u>molar triangle</u>. The character of this triangle is important to the dentist who practices endodontics. The MB orifice is well to the MB portion of the tooth, and the lingual orifice is also well to the lingual portion. However, the DB orifice is not so far buccally placed as the MB orifice, and, in fact, is located somewhat toward the distal surface. The lingual orifice has the largest diameter, and the DB the smallest.

5.   Mid Root Cross Section - The outlines of the three root branches are visible in a mid root cross section. The lingual root and its canal are the largest, and they are both ovoid, and wider mesiodistally. The MB root outline is also ovoid, but it is wider buccolingually, and when two canals are present, they are both circular. If one canal exists, it is normally ovoid and wider buccolingually similar to the root outline. The smallest root outline is that of the DB root, and it is less ovoid and more nearly round, as is its canal outline.

G.   Maxillary Second Molar:

The pulp cavity of this tooth is so similar to that of the first molar, that only the following differences will be described:

1.   There is not so much flare in the roots from any aspect, and consequently not so much spread in the root canals.

2.   Although the two facial roots are closer together, and sometimes even fused, there are still at least two complete root canals at the buccal.

3.   There is most often but one root canal in the MB root. However, this tooth's most common exception from normal is two canals in the MB root, similar to the normal anatomy of the first molar.

4.   Because the DL cusp is normally reduced in size, the DL pulp horn is also relatively smaller.

5.   When the general crown form of this tooth is heart shaped, the outline of the pulp chamber in a cervical line cross section is usually roughly triangular, as compared to the rhomboidal pattern most often seen.

H.   Maxillary Third Molar:

No standard pulp anatomy can be described for this tooth because of its wide variation in form, although the most common situation shows a typical maxillary molar configuration with three roots and three root canals. This tooth is normally a poor risk for root canal therapy.

I.   Mandibular Incisors:

1.   Introduction:

As with the maxillary incisors, the pulp cavities of the two mandibular incisors are so similar that they will be discussed together. Unlike the maxillary incisors, however, their pulpal outline is wider labiolingually. By far the majority (about 70-90%) of mandibular incisor (and canine) specimens exhibit the expected one root and one root canal. In rare instances (1-2%), these teeth reveal two fully formed canals, usually when the root is bifurcated. In the remaining cases, there is one canal which branches into two canals. When this occurs, the two branches may either reunite in the apical third to exit via a common foramen, or may remain separate, exiting through individual foramina. When there are two root canals present in any portion of the root, they are almost always labially and lingually located. The most common situation of a single root and canal will be described and diagrammed.

144

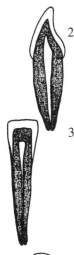

2. Labiolingual Section:

    a. Pulp chamber - From this aspect, the outline of the pulp chamber is similar to that of the maxillary incisors. It is pointed at the incisal, and widens to its largest diameter at about the mid cingulum level.

    b. Pulp canal - The canal is widest at the cervix, from where it tapers rather evenly to the single constricted foramen.

3. Mesiodistal Section:

    a. Pulp chamber - The chamber is generally narrower in this view than in the labiolingual section, and is much narrower when compared to the maxillary incisors. It is widest near the incisal limit, and then it narrows evenly to the cervical line. Unlike the maxillary incisors, the incisal limit lacks any pulp horns, and is flat or slightly rounded instead.

    b. Pulp canal - From the cervical line, the single canal tapers only slightly, but regularly, to the apical foramen.

4. Cervical Cross Section - At this level, the pulp outline is ovoid, and wider labiolingually than mesiodistally, just as is the root outline.

5. Mid Root Cross Section - Even though it is still ovoid, the canal is more constricted, and relatively narrower labiolingually than in the preceding view.

J. Mandibular Canine:

The pulp cavity of the mandibular canine is much like that of the maxillary canine, with the following exceptions:

1. The dimensions of the root canal are generally not quite so great.

2. Both the root and root canal outlines are narrower in the mesiodistal dimension, when compared to the maxillary canine.

3. Occasionally there are two roots, which are labially and lingually located, each with its own pulp canal. This phenomenon is difficult to diagnose, since routine x-rays tend to superimpose the labial and lingual roots and their canals.

4. The proportion of variations in canal numbers which was described for mandibular incisors also applies to mandibular canines, although one study indicated a greater number (as many as 6%) with two complete root canals.

K. Mandibular First Premolar:

1. Introduction:

The pulp cavity of this tooth is wider faciolingually than mesiodistally, and shows many other similarities to the mandibular canine.

2. Buccolingual Section:

    a. Pulp chamber - Normally, there are two pulp horns which correspond in size to the cusps of this tooth. There is a large and pointed buccal horn, and a small, sometimes rounded, lingual horn. However, it is not unusual for the lingual horn to be entirely missing, in which case the outline is like that of the canine. The widest point of the chamber is still near the cervical line, although it is wider toward the occlusal than is the outline of the canine.

    b. Pulp canal - From the cervical line, the single canal tapers rather evenly to the apical third, where it is constricted to its apical termination. Occasionally, there is a mid root branching into two canals, which reunite in the apical third. And, a few specimens exhibit a branching in the apical third, with two small foramina. Like the canine, a few teeth also have two roots and two root canals, facially and lingually oriented.

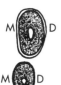

3. Mesiodistal Section - This section is nearly identical to the mandibular canine, although the canine has a longer root, and hence a longer pulp canal.

4. Cervical Cross Section - Both root and root canal in this view are normally ovoid, and wider buccolingually.

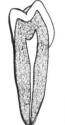

5. Mid Root Cross Section - In this section, the canal outline is normally round.

L. Mandibular Second Premolar:

The mandibular second premolar is similar to the first premolar except:

1. The lingual pulp horn is normally larger to correspond to the larger lingual cusp(s). Some Y type specimens exhibit two lingual pulp horns.

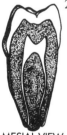

2. The root and root canal cross sections are more often ovoid, wider buccolingually, than round.

3. The pulp chamber is relatively wider buccolingually than mesiodistally, when compared to the first premolar.

4. In the buccolingual section, the separation of the pulp chamber and canal is normally distinguishable, as contrasted to the more regular taper in the first premolar.

Linguobuccal Section
Distal View

5. The second premolar root, and thus its root canal, are slightly longer.

M. Mandibular First Molar:

1. Introduction:

Although mandibular first molars normally possess two roots, they exhibit three root canals about 70% of the time. Two of these canals are found in the mesial root (MB and ML), while the distal root contains only one canal. In a majority of the remaining 30% of the cases, there are four canals with two per root. In some cases, however, there is only one canal in each root, or a total of two canals. The most common situation of three canals will be discussed and diagrammed. The buccolingual dimension of the pulp chamber is less than the mesiodistal dimension, corresponding to the crown dimensions.

2. Buccolingual Section:

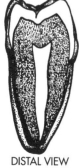

a. Mesial aspect (chamber and canals) - There are two pulp horns (MB and ML) of nearly equal size and pointedness, corresponding to the two mesial cusps. The chamber is widest near the pulp horn level, but constricts only slightly to the chamber floor, which is apical to the cervical line.

The mesial root is larger than the distal, and it is the only one visible in this section. The mesial root normally has two root canals, named MB and ML canals. They constrict only a little from the chamber floor to their separate foramina. In some cases, there is only one canal, which is quite wide buccolingually. Also, on occasion, the two canals unite in the apical third, and share a common foramen.

MESIAL VIEW

b. Distal aspect (chamber and canal) - The outline of the chamber is generally smaller but otherwise looks like it did from the mesial aspect, except that a slight pulp horn, corresponding to the distal cusp, can sometimes be seen. The DB and DL pulp horns are about the same size.

There is normally a single canal, which is quite wide buccolingually, and tapers evenly to the apex. It is much larger than either of the mesial canals. As previously mentioned, it is not uncommon to find two canals, similar to those of the mesial root.

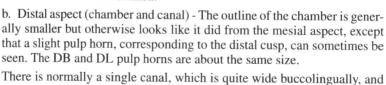

DISTAL VIEW

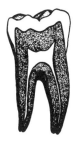

3. Mesiodistal Section (Buccal Aspect):

    a. Pulp chamber - The chamber is widest at the pulp horn level, and constricts slightly to its floor, which is apical to the cervical line. Normally, only the two buccal pulp horns can be seen, but occasionally a small distal horn is also visible in the newly erupted specimen. The MB pulp horn is noticeably larger than the DB horn.

    b. Pulp canals - Only two canals are visible from either the buccal or lingual aspect. The distal canal is visible from both aspects. However, of the two mesial canals, only the MB canal is visible from the buccal aspect, and the ML canal is only visible from the lingual aspect. There is also more spread to the canals in this section, when compared to a mesial view.

4. Cervical Line Cross Section - The outline of a cervical cross section follows the crown's external contour. There is usually evidence of all five cusps in the form of rounded humps at the five points of the roughly pentagonal outline. The floor of the chamber, apical to the cervical line, exhibits three orifices, two mesially placed, and one distally located. The distal is the largest, and it is quite wide buccolingually, while the two mesial orifices are usually circular.

5. Mid Root Cross Section - There are normally two roots, both of which are wider buccolingually. The mesial root, which is somewhat kidney shaped, is the largest, and contains the two more or less circular root canal outlines, of which the MB is slightly larger in diameter. The smaller distal root contains one large ovoid canal, which is wider buccolingually, like the root shape. In some cases, the distal root outline, and even the root canal, may exhibit a kidney shape.

N. Mandibular Second Molar:

The pulp cavity of the second molar is similar to that of the first molar, with the following exceptions:

    1. There are still normally two root canals in the mesial root, but more often than in the first molar, there is only one. There is likewise an even smaller chance of two root canals in the distal root.

    2. The pulp chamber is generally not as large, and the two mesial orifices are located closer together.

    3. In a buccolingual section, the two mesial canals are not as divergent.

    4. There is almost never a distal pulp horn.

O. Mandibular Third Molar:

Like the maxillary third molar, no standard pulp outline can be described, due to the wide variation in form. However, most common is the typical mandibular molar configuration of two roots and three root canals. Like the maxillary third molar, this tooth is normally a poor risk for root canal therapy.

PULP CHAMBER ANATOMY & COMPONENTS

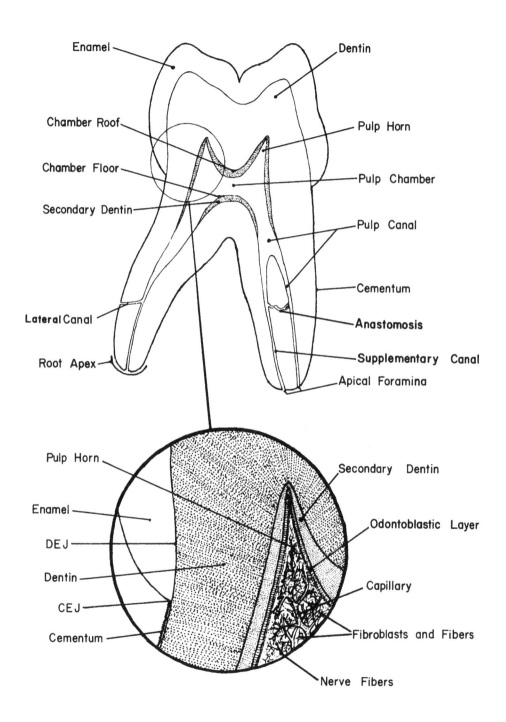

Enamel

Dentin

Chamber Roof

Pulp Horn

Chamber Floor

Pulp Chamber

Secondary Dentin

Pulp Canal

Cementum

Lateral Canal

Anastomosis

Root Apex

Supplementary Canal

Apical Foramina

Pulp Horn

Secondary Dentin

Enamel

Odontoblastic Layer

DEJ

Dentin

Capillary

CEJ

Cementum

Fibroblasts and Fibers

Nerve Fibers

148

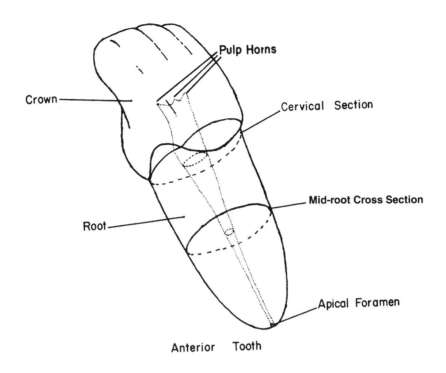

Pulp Horns

Crown

Cervical Section

Mid-root Cross Section

Root

Apical Foramen

Anterior   Tooth

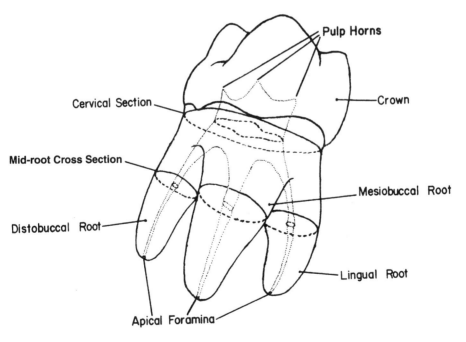

Pulp Horns

Cervical Section

Crown

Mid-root Cross Section

Mesiobuccal Root

Distobuccal Root

Lingual Root

Apical Foramina

Posterior   Tooth

EXAMPLES OF TOOTH SECTIONS

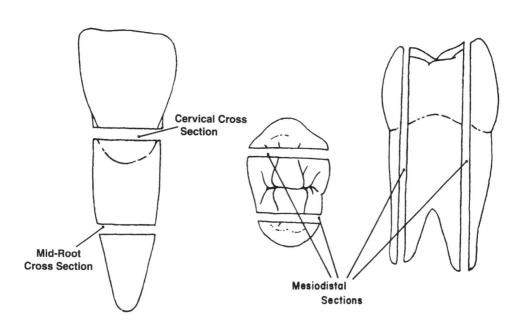

Cervical Cross Section

Mid-Root Cross Section

Mesiodistal Sections

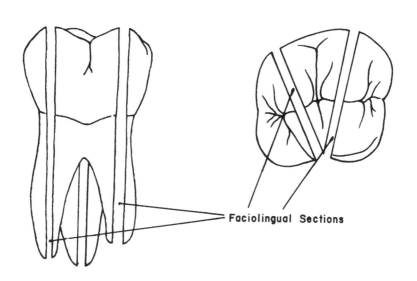

Faciolingual Sections

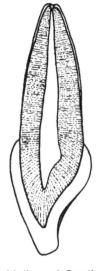

Labiolingual Section
Mesial View

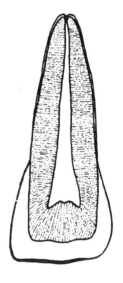

Mesiodistal Section
Lingual View

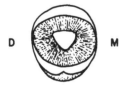

Cervical Section

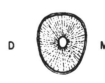

Mid-Root Section

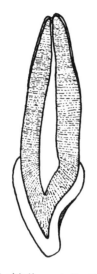

Labiolingual Section
Mesial View

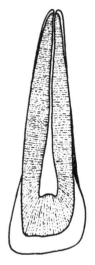

Mesiodistal Section
Lingual View

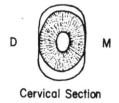

Cervical Section

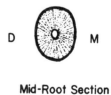

Mid-Root Section

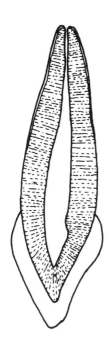

Labiolingual Section
Mesial View

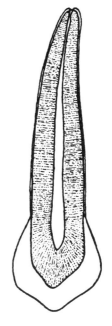

Mesiodistal Section
Lingual View

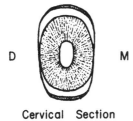

D   M

Cervical   Section

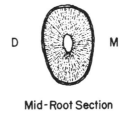

D   M

Mid-Root Section

MAXILLARY RIGHT FIRST PREMOLAR

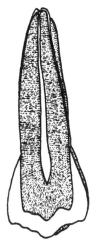

Distomesial Section
Buccal View

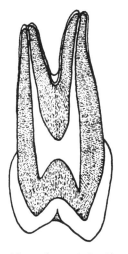

Linguobuccal Section
Distal View

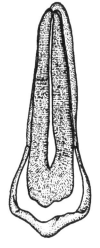

Mesiodistal Section
Lingual View

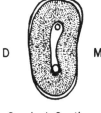

D   M

Cervical Section

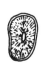

Single

2-roots

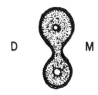

D   M

Laminated Mid-Root Section

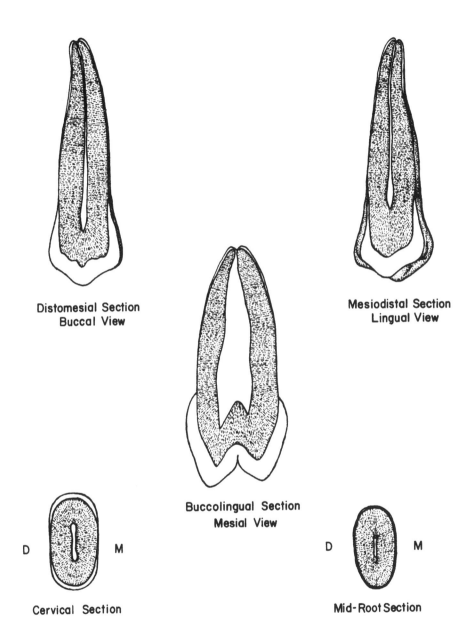

Distomesial Section
Buccal View

Mesiodistal Section
Lingual View

Buccolingual Section
Mesial View

D   M

Cervical Section

D   M

Mid-Root Section

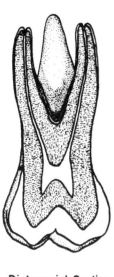

Distomesial Section
Buccal View

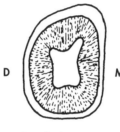

D   M

Cervical Section

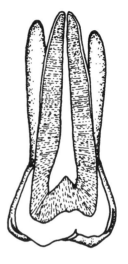

Mesiodistal Section
Lingual View

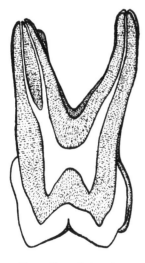

Buccolingual Section
Mesial View

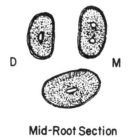

D   M

Mid-Root Section

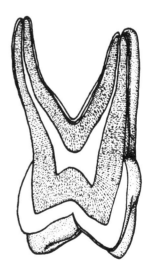

Linguobuccal Section
Distal View

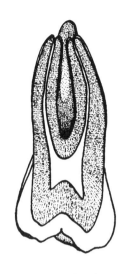

Distomesial Section
Buccal View

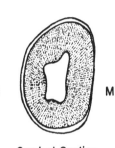

D   M

Cervical Section

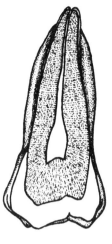

Mesiodistal Section
Lingual View

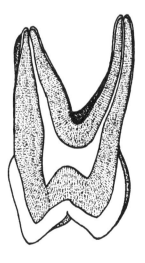

Buccolingual Section
Mesial View

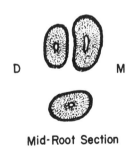

D   M

Mid-Root Section

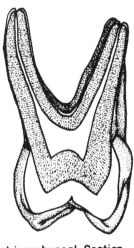

Linguobuccal Section
Distal View

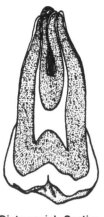

Distomesial Section
Buccal View

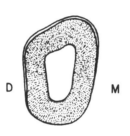

Cervical Section

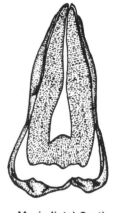

Mesiodistal Section
Lingual View

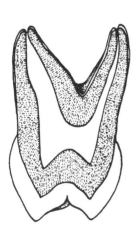

Buccolingual Section
Mesial View

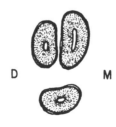

Mid-Root Section

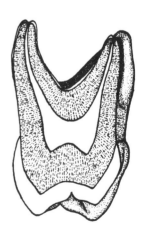

Linguobuccal Section
Distal View

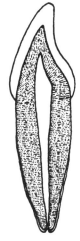

Labiolingual Section
Mesial View

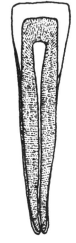

Mesiodistal Section
Lingual View

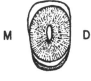

M   D

Cervical Section

M   D

Mid-Root Section

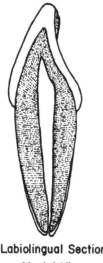

Labiolingual Section
Mesial View

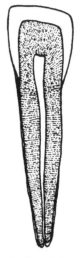

Mesiodistal Section
Lingual View

Cervical Section

Mid-Root Section

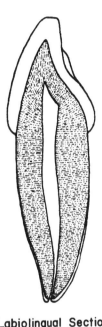

Labiolingual Section
Mesial View

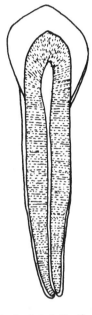

Mesiodistal Section
Lingual View

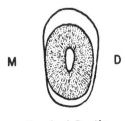

M   D

Cervical Section

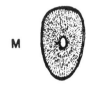

M   D

Mid-Root Section

MANDIBULAR RIGHT FIRST PREMOLAR

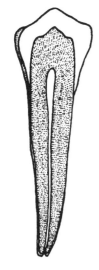

Distomesial Section
Buccal View

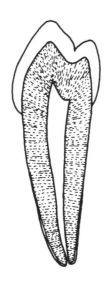

Buccolingual Section
Mesial View

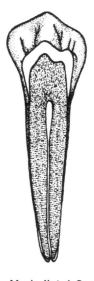

Mesiodistal Section
Lingual View

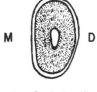

M   D

Cervical Section

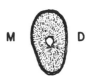

M   D

Mid-Root Section

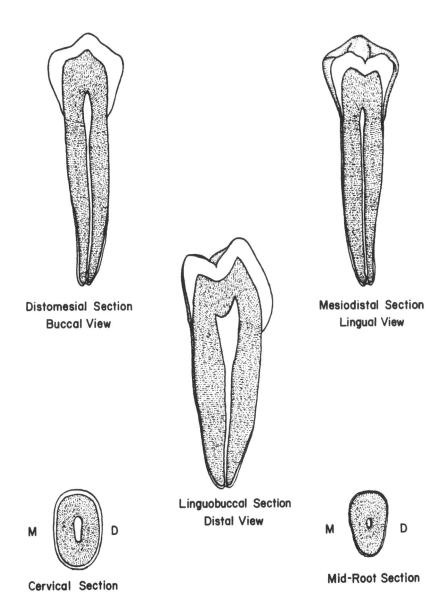

Distomesial Section
Buccal View

Mesiodistal Section
Lingual View

Linguobuccal Section
Distal View

M   D

Cervical Section

M   D

Mid-Root Section

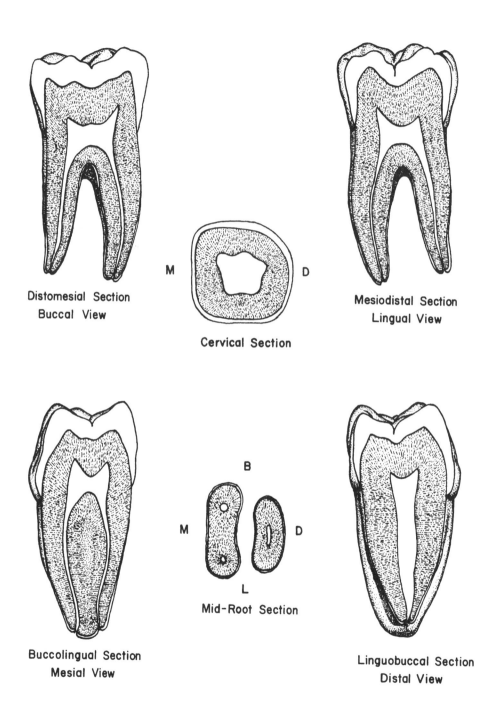

Distomesial Section
Buccal View

Cervical Section

M   D

Mesiodistal Section
Lingual View

Buccolingual Section
Mesial View

B

M   D

L

Mid-Root Section

Linguobuccal Section
Distal View

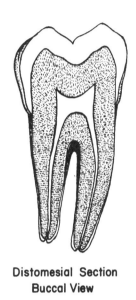

Distomesial Section
Buccal View

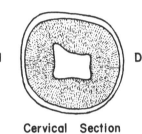

M   D

Cervical Section

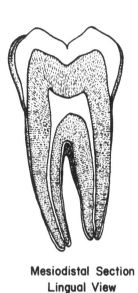

Mesiodistal Section
Lingual View

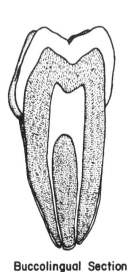

Buccolingual Section
Mesial View

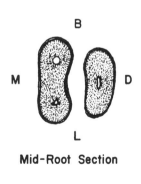

B

M   D

L

Mid-Root Section

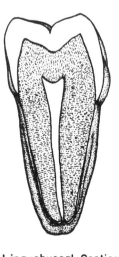

Linguobuccal Section
Distal View

MANDIBULAR RIGHT THIRD MOLAR

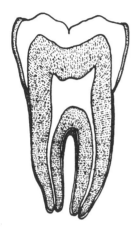

Distomesial Section
Buccal View

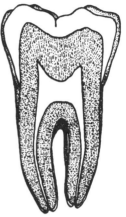

Mesiodistal Section
Lingual View

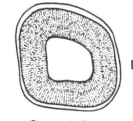

M   D

Cervical Section

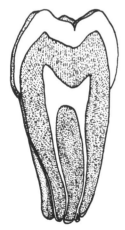

Buccolingual Section
Mesial View

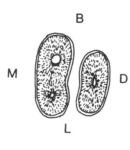

B

M   D

L

Mid-Root Section

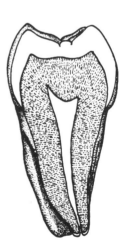

Linguobuccal Section
Distal View

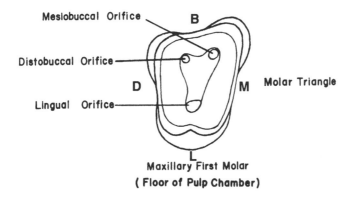

Mesiobuccal Orifice

Distobuccal Orifice

Lingual Orifice

B

D

M

L

Molar Triangle

Maxillary First Molar
(Floor of Pulp Chamber)

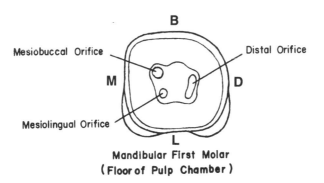

Mesiobuccal Orifice

Distal Orifice

M

D

Mesiolingual Orifice

B

L

Mandibular First Molar
(Floor of Pulp Chamber)

167

UNIT # 10

I. **Reading Assignment:**

Unit # 10 (The Deciduous Dentition)

II. **Specific Objectives:**

At the completion of this unit, the student will be able to:

A. Demonstrate a knowledge of the general differences between the permanent and deciduous teeth, by describing them, or selecting the correct response from a list, when given one or more differences, or any appropriate implications of these differences.

B. Demonstrate a knowledge of the morphology of each surface of the crown and root of all deciduous teeth by:

1. describing,

2. selecting the correct information from a list,

3. or interpreting a diagram to identify or name any of the following features:

a. Contours of any surface, or margin of any surface.

b. Structural entities such as grooves, pits, ridges, cusps, fossae, etc.

c. Relative dimensions and shape.

d. Root numbers, location, and contours.

e. Any other surface feature.

Furthermore, the student will be able to make comparisons of any of these features between any of the deciduous teeth.

C. Make comparisons between specific deciduous teeth and their permanent counterparts, where appropriate, by describing the differences, or selecting the correct information from a list.

D. Determine from a diagram or description which deciduous tooth is being described, or illustrated.

E. Provide the correct universal number or Palmer notation for a given diagram or description of any deciduous tooth.

The student is also responsible for any material which was to have been mastered in previous units.

UNIT # 10
THE DECIDUOUS DENTITION

I. **Introduction:**

A. Until this point in the text, the deciduous dentition has assumed the status of a second class citizen. Even though the time spent studying the deciduous teeth will be less than that devoted to the permanent teeth, they are nonetheless important.

B. Until a generation or two ago, most parents were guilty of disregarding the value of the deciduous teeth of their children. But even worse, many dentists like-wise took this view. As a result, the primary teeth were considered as simply a tem-porary phase in the more important process of acquiring a permanent dentition. Rarely did these teeth receive adequate attention, and the customary treatment was extraction of any deciduous tooth which became so diseased it caused dysfunction or pain to the child. One of the most common consequences of this philosophy of treatment (or lack of it) was a loss of space with the potential for crowding and malocclusion in the permanent dentition. Fortunately, attitudes have changed and the dental profession, along with the general public, now have a more realistic ap-preciation of the value of the primary teeth.

C. As previously indicated, there are a total of twenty deciduous teeth, ten per arch, and five per quadrant. In each quadrant, there are two deciduous incisors and one canine, just as in the anterior segment of the permanent dentition. However, unlike the permanent posterior teeth, there are no premolars, and only two molars per quadrant. Deciduous teeth exhibit a functional role similar to their permanent counterparts.

D. A brief review of those portions of the introductory unit which concern the deciduous dentition would be of value to the student. It should also be noted that the development and life cycle of the deciduous teeth will be discussed in the succeed-ing unit.

II. **Comparisons Between Permanent and Deciduous Teeth:**

A. External Considerations:

1. The deciduous teeth are generally smaller than their permanent counter-parts. This size disparity exists for crown and root portions of both anterior and posterior teeth.

2. The crown portion of the deciduous teeth is quite short inciso (occluso) gingivally, relative to its total crown-root length, when contrasted to the same dimensions of permanent teeth.

3. The crowns of deciduous teeth are wider mesiodistally, relative to their inciso (occluso) gingival height, when compared to the same dimensions of permanent teeth.

4. The crowns of deciduous teeth are more constricted faciolingually at the cervical line than are those of permanent teeth.

5. Because of a greater occlusal convergence of the buccal and lingual sur-faces, the occlusal tables of deciduous molars are relatively more constricted faciolingually than are the crowns of permanent molars.

6. There is a cervical ridge on both labial and lingual surfaces of deciduous anterior teeth, as well as on the buccal surface of deciduous posterior teeth. This ridge is normally much more prominent than any analogous structure found on permanent molars.

7. In comparison to the crown height occlusocervically, the roots of decidu-ous molars are relatively longer than those of permanent molars. They are, how-

169

ever, less substantial in their other dimensions, which in summary makes them longer and thinner.

8.   The roots of deciduous molars reveal much more flare, or spreading, than do roots of the permanent molars. This flare creates additional space for the permanent premolar crown to develop. Their greater spread, coupled with the more slender shape and lack of a root trunk, make deciduous molar roots easier to fracture during extraction procedures.

9.   The roots of deciduous molars branch almost directly from the base of the crown, so that there is no easily identifiable root trunk, as there is in the permanent molars. This feature also creates more space for the developing permanent premolar crown.

10.   The crowns of deciduous teeth are lighter in color. This is because they are more opaque and thus exhibit a whitish-white or even bluish-white cast, compared to the yellowish and grayish-white shades of permanent tooth crowns.

B.   Internal Considerations:

1.   The enamel in the crowns of deciduous teeth is relatively thin, when compared to permanent teeth.

2.   The dentin of primary teeth is also relatively thin, in comparison to permanent teeth.

3. The pulp cavity is relatively larger in the deciduous teeth. The mesial pulp horns of deciduous molars are especially large.

III. Description of Individual Deciduous Teeth:

Instead of describing the deciduous teeth in as much detail as the permanent teeth, greater use of comparisons will be made.

A.   Maxillary Central Incisor:

1.   General considerations - The deciduous maxillary central incisor is similar in many respects to its permanent successor. It has the same arch position, function, and relative shape. In addition to the previously elicited general differences, there are two major specific contrasts to the permanent maxillary central. First, there are no mamelons in newly erupted teeth. Second, this is the only anterior tooth of either dentition, in which the mesiodistal crown width is normally greater than the incisocervical crown height.

2.   Labial aspect - The mesial and distal outlines are more convex than in the permanent central. The generally convex labial surface is smooth, and rarely exhibits developmental depressions or imbrication lines. The incisal outline is relatively flat, lacks mamelons, and usually slopes toward the distal after wear. The distoincisal angle is slightly more rounded than the mesioincisal angle. The cervical line curves evenly toward the root.

3.   Lingual aspect - The cingulum is more prominent, and extends farther incisally than on the permanent tooth. The marginal ridges are also more prominent, and the fossa is deeper.

4.   Mesial aspect - The mesial surface is similar to that of the permanent tooth, except that in the deciduous tooth it is relatively wider labiolingually, and the cervical line exhibits less curvature incisally.

5.   Distal aspect - The distal is similar to the mesial aspect, except that the cervical line curvature is less.

6.   Incisal aspect - The almost straight incisal edge divides the crown into roughly equal labial and lingual portions. The most noticeable feature, however, is the crown's relatively great mesiodistal width.

7. Root - The single root is generally round and tapers evenly to the apex. It is longer, relative to crown length, than in the permanent central.

B. Maxillary Lateral Incisor:

This tooth will not be described in detail, since it is so similar to the central incisor; only the following differences will be pointed out:

1. The deciduous lateral incisor is smaller than the central in all dimensions. However, unlike the central, the crown of the lateral incisor is wider incisocervically than mesiodistally.

2. Both incisal angles display greater rounding, with the distoincisal angle more so than the mesioincisal.

3. The marginal ridges on the lingual surface are more prominent, with a resultant deeper lingual fossa.

4. From the incisal aspect, the much narrower mesiodistal dimension is reflected in an outline which is more rhomboidal and more convex.

5. The root outlines are similar, but the lateral's root is relatively longer, and its apex is not so rounded.

C. Maxillary Canine:

1. General considerations - The deciduous maxillary canine exhibits a crown which is also quite wide mesiodistally. However, this dimension is slightly less than the incisocervical measurement.

2. Labial aspect - Like the deciduous maxillary incisors, the mesial and distal outlines bulge convexly to the cervical line. The height of contour of these margins is found at the level of the contact area. Interestingly, the mesial and distal contact areas are located at the same level incisocervically, rather than at different levels, as in the permanent canine. This feature is also true for the deciduous mandibular canine. Before incisal wear, the cusp is relatively more prominent than that of the permanent tooth. The mesioincisal slope is normally longer than the distoincisal slope, especially after attrition. The cervical line exhibits an even curvature apically. Normally, no developmental depressions or imbrication lines are present.

3. Lingual aspect - The cingulum is quite prominent, as are the lingual ridge and marginal ridges. Normally, ML and DL fossae are present. Unlike the permanent canine, there is occasionally a tubercle located where the cingulum merges with the lingual ridge near the center of the lingual surface.

4. Mesial aspect - This surface is similar to the primary maxillary incisors, except that labiolingually the tooth is thicker, and the cervical line depth is less.

5. Distal aspect - The distal surface is similar to the mesial, except that the cervical line shows less curvature.

6. Incisal aspect - From this aspect, the outline is rhomboidal, but has more rounding than the permanent canine exhibits. The cusp tip is offset to the distal, and thus the mesial cusp ridge is longer.

7. Root - From all aspects, the root is similar to the deciduous maxillary incisor roots, except that it is longer.

D. Maxillary First Molar:

1. General considerations - This tooth's crown does not resemble any other primary or permanent molar crown, but does exhibit some similarities to the crowns of permanent premolars. However, the root form is typical of maxillary molars. Like all permanent maxillary posterior teeth, the crown

171

shows its greatest dimension buccolingually. The occlusal table reveals only two prominent cusps, the MB and ML cusps. The two distal cusps, and especially the DL cusp, are greatly diminished. This feature creates the most conspicuous comparison to a permanent maxillary premolar crown.

2. Buccal aspect - The mesiodistal diameter is much greater than the crown height. The mesial and distal outlines are convex, and constrict greatly toward the cervix from the heights of contour, which are located at the contact areas near the junction of the occlusal and middle thirds. The occlusal outline is comparatively straight, since the two buccal cusps are nowhere near as prominent or sharp as in the permanent maxillary molars. An essential difference from the permanent tooth is found in the contour of the cervical line, since its depth of curvature is much greater toward the mesial than the distal, thus giving the crown the appearance of being offset toward the mesial. The entire surface is relatively smooth and lacks grooves or depressions. Occlusally, the buccal surface is mostly flat, but in the gingival third the cervical ridge is prominent, especially the mesial portion. The surface has a crest of curvature in the cervical third.

3. Lingual aspect - The lingual outline is much like that of the buccal view, but with a lessened mesiodistal dimension. The account of the mesial and distal margins parallels their description for the buccal surface. Even though the ML cusp is not very tall, it is quite bulky and dominates the occlusal outline. The DL cusp is so diminutive that the DB cusp is also partially visible from this aspect. Unlike the buccal surface, the cervical line is evenly, and slightly, curved toward the apex. The lingual surface is generally convex and smooth without grooves or depressions. The height of contour is more cervically located, at about the middle and cervical third junction, as compared to its middle third location in permanent maxillary posterior teeth.

4. Mesial aspect - The disparity between the faciolingual widths of this surface at its cervical and occlusal margins is much more than in the permanent maxillary molars. Cervically, the dimension is considerably wider, due to the prominent cervical ridge on the buccal, as well as the greater taper of the buccal and lingual outlines toward the occlusal. The buccal outline is dominated by the cervical ridge and crest of curvature in the cervical third. The remainder of the buccal outline is usually straight, or even slightly concave. The lingual outline is generally convex, but with a more cervically located crest of curvature than is present on the permanent molars. The two mesial cusps and the mesial marginal ridge make up the occlusal outline. From this aspect, the ML cusp is more generous in height and size than is the MB cusp. Because of the diminished buccolingual dimension at the occlusal, the marginal ridge is relatively short. The cervical line is slightly curved toward the occlusal.

5. Distal aspect - The distal surface itself is considerably smaller than the mesial surface. Since the buccal surface tapers toward the distal, much of it is visible from this aspect. The DB cusp is more prominent than the minute DL cusp, and the distal marginal ridge is less pronounced than is the mesial. The mesial cusps actually provide the occlusal outline from this aspect. The cervical ridge is not so prominent in the buccal outline as it is from the mesial aspect. The cervical line is straight to slightly curved occlusally.

6. Occlusal aspect - The general shape of this tooth from the occlusal aspect is an unusual five sided figure. The crown dimensions are less buccolingually toward the distal, and less mesiodistally toward the lingual.

a. Cusps - Like most permanent maxillary molars, there are four cusps, but in reality the two distal cusps are so meager that there is a closer similarity to a premolar occlusal table. The ML cusp is the bulkiest, and also the longest, while the DL cusp is the smallest, and on occasion, is entirely absent. Of the two remaining cusps, the MB is of greater proportions than the DB. In fact, the lingual cusp ridge of the MB cusp is the most prominent single elevation within the occlusal table.

b. Transverse ridge - A very prominent transverse ridge dominates the occlusal table of this tooth, and like the permanent maxillary molars, consists of the lingual cusp ridge of the MB cusp and the buccal cusp ridge of the ML cusp.

c. Oblique ridge - The majority of specimens exhibit an oblique ridge, extending from the ML cusp to the DB cusp, similar to, but not as prominent as the analogous structure of permanent molars.

d. Fossae - This tooth contains three fossae: a well defined central fossa, plus mesial and distal triangular fossae.

e. Pits and grooves - There are mesial and distal pits, which are located in the depth of their respective triangular fossae. There is also a central pit, with a central groove connecting it with the mesial and distal pits. The buccal groove, which also originates in the central pit, extends buccally, separating the MB and DB cusps on the occlusal surface only. The distal triangular fossa also contains a disto-occlusal groove, which extends obliquely on the occlusal table, and parallels the oblique ridge just distal to it. This groove rarely crosses onto the lingual surface like the distolingual groove of the permanent maxillary molars does.

7. Roots - As previously pointed out, deciduous molars possess no root trunk, and the root branches are more slender, and reveal greater flare. Otherwise, the root structure of the first molar exhibits three root branches which are similar in name, location, and general contours, to those of the permanent maxillary molars. The lingual root is the largest and longest, followed in size by the MB root, and the DB root, respectively.

E. Maxillary Second Molar:

There is really no need to describe this tooth in detail, since, despite the general differences between deciduous and permanent molars, it closely resembles the permanent maxillary first molar. So, other than those general differences, its contours, occlusal pattern, and roots are modeled after the permanent tooth. In fact, this tooth even exhibits at least a trace of the cusp of Carabelli trait in most specimens.

F. Mandibular Central Incisor:

1. General considerations - This tooth bears a much closer resemblance to the deciduous mandibular lateral incisor than it does to its permanent counterpart, or to any deciduous maxillary incisor. The mandibular central incisor crown is symmetrical, when viewed from the labial, lingual, or incisal, just like its permanent successor. In relation to its incisogingival height, the crown is relatively wider mesiodistally than in permanent incisors. However, the mesiodistal dimension is not greater than the incisocervical dimension, as it is in the deciduous maxillary central incisor.

2. Labial aspect - The mesial and distal outlines are evenly convex from the sharp mesioincisal and distoincisal angles to the cervical line. The convexity is less than that exhibited by the deciduous maxillary incisors. The height of contour of these margins is at the contact area in the incisal third. The incisal margin is straight, and devoid of mamelons. The labial surface itself is smooth,

lacking developmental depressions, and generally is flatter than the labial surface of permanent incisors.

3. Lingual aspect - The cingulum is well defined, but the marginal ridges are not so well developed as in the maxillary incisors, thus outlining a lingual fossa which is quite shallow. All margins are comparable to those of the facial surface.

4. Mesial aspect - From this view of the crown, the most outstanding feature is the relatively greater labiolingual width, when compared to the permanent incisors. The incisal edge is located over the root center, and the cervical line contour is evenly curved toward the incisal.

5. Distal aspect - The distal surface is similar to the mesial, except that the cervical line exhibits less depth of curvature.

6. Incisal aspect - From this view, the incisal edge is straight, and it divides the labial and lingual portions of the crown into nearly equal halves. The mesiodistal and labiolingual dimensions are nearly equal, whereas in the maxillary central incisor, the crown was noticeably wider mesiodistally. As in the permanent tooth, mesial and distal portions of the crown are symmetrical from this aspect.

7. Root - The root is single, relatively long, and slender. The labial and lingual surfaces are convex, while the mesial and distal surfaces are somewhat flattened.

G. Mandibular Lateral Incisor:

This tooth is similar in form to the deciduous mandibular central incisor, with the following exceptions:

1. The crown is slightly longer incisogingivally and wider mesiodistally.

2. From the labial or lingual aspect, the incisal outline slopes slightly toward the distal, with a resultant distoincisal angle which is more rounded, as is the distal margin of the crown. The distal margin is also a little shorter.

3. The cingulum and marginal ridges are usually a little larger, and the lingual fossa is a little deeper.

4. From the incisal, the crown is not quite symmetrical like the central, since the cingulum bulges toward the distal, as it does in the permanent mandibular lateral.

5. The root may present a distal curvature in its apical third, and it normally has at least a distal longitudinal groove.

H. Mandibular Canine:

In general form, this tooth resembles the deciduous maxillary canine, but its relative dimensions are somewhat different. The most notable contrasts with the maxillary canine reveal that:

1. The mandibular canine is a much narrower tooth labiolingually, and this is the crown dimension in which the two teeth differ most.

2. The mesiodistal width of the mandibular canine is also considerably less than that of the maxillary canine. The incisocervical dimension of the two deciduous canines is the same. Therefore, the crown of the mandibular canine has an incisocervical height which is noticeably greater than its mesiodistal width, while these two dimensions of the maxillary canine are much closer to being equal.

3. The distoincisal slope is longer on the mandibular canine, whereas on the maxillary canine it is the mesioincisal slope which is longer.

4. The cingulum, marginal ridges, and cervical ridges are less pronounced on the crown of the mandibular canine.

5. The mandibular canine root is shorter.

I. Mandibular First Molar:

1. General considerations - This tooth has a crown unlike any other primary or permanent tooth. However, it does have two roots which are positioned similarly to those of the other primary and permanent mandibular molars. Its crown is wider mesiodistally than buccolingually, as is characteristic of all mandibular molars of both dentitions.

2. Buccal aspect - The mesial outline is uniquely straight occlusogingivally for most of its length, but the distal outline is convex, and overhangs the cervical line. The occlusal outline reveals two buccal cusps, of which the MB cusp is much larger. From this view, the cusp outlines are more prominent than those of the deciduous maxillary first molar. There is a depression separating the two buccal cusp outlines, but rarely does the buccal groove extend onto the buccal surface in the depression. The cervical line is deeper, and offset toward the mesial, just like it is on the deciduous maxillary first molar. The cervical ridge is also quite prominent, especially in the mesial portion.

3. Lingual aspect - The lingual surface is shorter occlusocervically than the buccal surface. It is also smooth and convex, and lacks any depressions or ridges. The mesial and distal margins are similar to those of the buccal aspect, but the cervical outline is rather straight, unlike the buccal aspect where it is irregular and has a deep offset to the mesial. The occlusal outline shows two lingual cusps, of which the ML cusp is larger and sharper. Portions of the two buccal cusps can also be seen.

4. Mesial aspect - The most striking feature, from this view, is the cervical ridge representing the crest of curvature in the gingival third of the buccal outline. Both mesial cusps are visible. The contact area is located near the junction of the occlusal and middle thirds, but the height of contour is difficult to pinpoint because of the flatness of the surface. The cervical line is located farther cervically on the buccal, and extends to a more occlusal level at the lingual.

5. Distal aspect - All four cusps can be seen from this aspect, with the MB cusp the longest. The distal marginal ridge is much less prominent than the mesial, and is located at a more cervical level. The cervical line is relatively straight, and located at the same level on both the buccal and lingual, in contrast to its appearance on the mesial surface.

6. Occlusal aspect - The general shape of the occlusal table is somewhat rectangular, if the bulging of the cervical ridge at the mesiobuccal is disregarded. Typical of mandibular molars, the crown is wider mesiodistally.

a. Cusps - The four cusps, from largest to smallest in size, are the MB, ML, DB, DL. Actually, the two mesial cusps are considerably larger than the distal cusps, as was the case on the crown of the maxillary first molar.

b. Transverse ridge - The buccal cusp ridge of the ML cusp and the lingual cusp ridge of the MB cusp form a prominent transverse ridge.

c. Fossae - The same three fossae are present as are found on the deciduous maxillary first molar, and they are the central fossa, and mesial and distal triangular fossae.

d. Pits and grooves - There are normally only two pits. The central pit is the deepest pit, and is located in the central fossa, which is toward the distal margin, rather than centrally located, as its name might imply. The mesial pit is located in the depth of the mesial triangular fossa. The central groove crosses the transverse ridge and connects the mesial and central pits. Since there is usually no distal pit, the central pit is normally the central groove's distal termination. The buccal groove also originates in the central pit, and extends buccally to fade out on the occlusal surface between the two buccal cusps. The third groove to originate in the central pit is the lingual groove, which extends lingually and separates the two lingual cusps. It also fades out before exiting the occlusal surface.

7.   Roots - The mesial and distal roots have a location similar to those of permanent mandibular molars. Both roots are widest buccolingually, but the mesial root is longer and much wider than the distal root. The apex of the mesial root is normally flat, almost to the point of being square buccolingually, a fact which is unique to this particular tooth. The shorter distal root has a more rounded apex. Both proximal surfaces of the mesial root usually exhibit root concavities. Of course, the general differences which were previously outlined between primary and permanent molar roots apply to this tooth.

J.   Mandibular Second Molar:

Disregarding size, and the general differences between deciduous and permanent molars, this tooth so closely resembles the permanent mandibular first molar, that it will not be necessary to describe it in detail. Major differences include the following:

1.   The MB, DB, and distal cusps are more nearly equal in size on the deciduous tooth.

2.   The occlusal table is relatively narrower buccolingually and less pentagonal than that of the permanent first molar.

3.   The mesial root is longer and wider than the distal root on the deciduous tooth, whereas they were of about equal length on the permanent first molar.

IV.   Pulp Cavities: Deciduous Teeth

As pointed out, the pulp cavities, and especially the pulp chambers and pulp horns, are relatively larger in the deciduous teeth. No detailed description of the pulp cavities for individual deciduous teeth will be offered. Endodontia is rarely attempted for primary teeth.

V.   Conclusion:

A large segment of material concerning development of the deciduous dentition was excluded from this unit, and will be presented in the final unit.

MAXILLARY RIGHT DECIDUOUS CENTRAL INCISOR

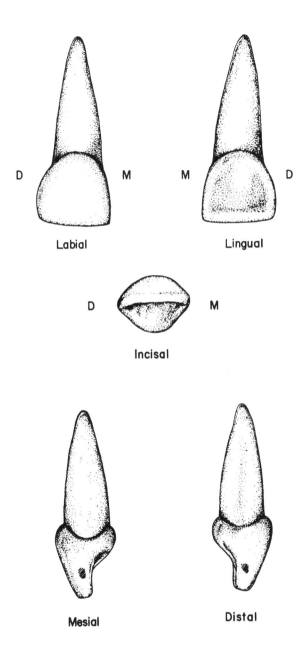

D   M

Labial

M   D

Lingual

D   M

Incisal

Mesial

Distal

MAXILLARY RIGHT DECIDUOUS LATERAL INCISOR

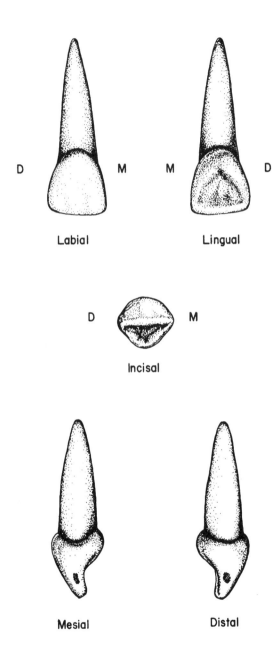

D   M   M   D

Labial   Lingual

D   M

Incisal

Mesial   Distal

MAXILLARY RIGHT DECIDUOUS CANINE

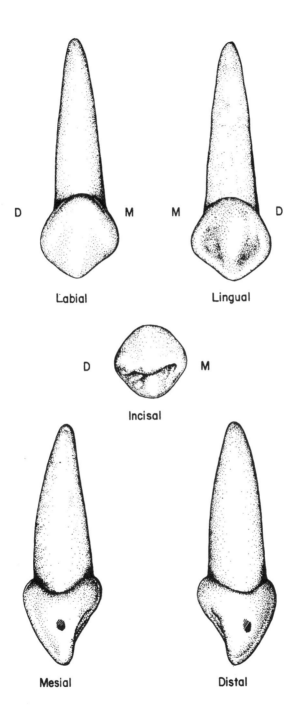

D M   M D

Labial   Lingual

D M

Incisal

Mesial   Distal

MAXILLARY RIGHT DECIDUOUS FIRST MOLAR

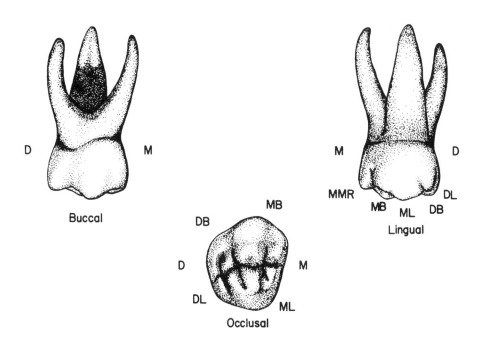

Buccal

Occlusal

Lingual

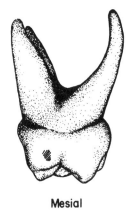

Mesial

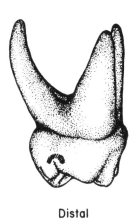

Distal

ML - Mesiolingual Cusp
DL - Distolingual Cusp
DB - Distobuccal Cusp
MB - Mesiobuccal Cusp
MMR - Mesial Marginal Ridge

180

MAXILLARY RIGHT DECIDUOUS SECOND MOLAR

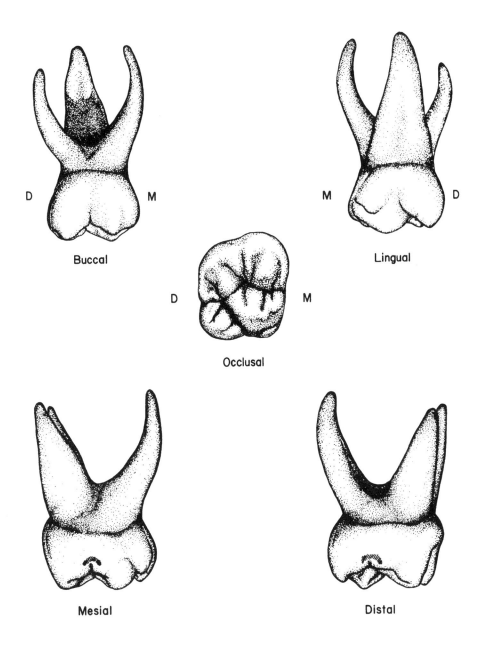

D   M
Buccal

M   D
Lingual

D   M
Occlusal

Mesial

Distal

181

MANDIBULAR RIGHT DECIDUOUS CENTRAL INCISOR

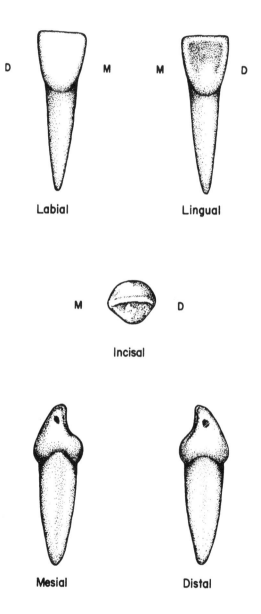

D M Labial

M D Lingual

M D Incisal

Mesial Distal

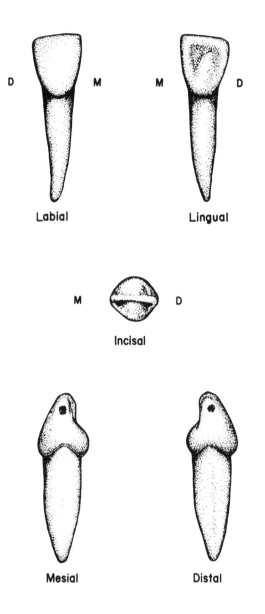

Labial

Lingual

Incisal

Mesial

Distal

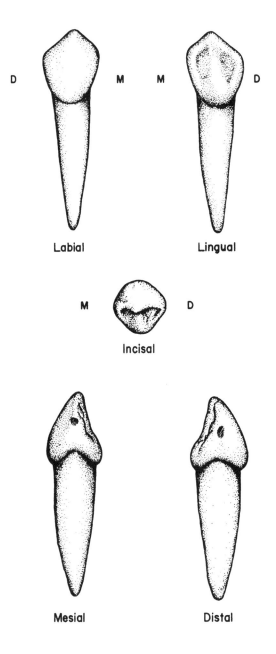

D　M　M　D

Labial　Lingual

M　D

Incisal

Mesial　Distal

MANDIBULAR RIGHT DECIDUOUS FIRST MOLAR

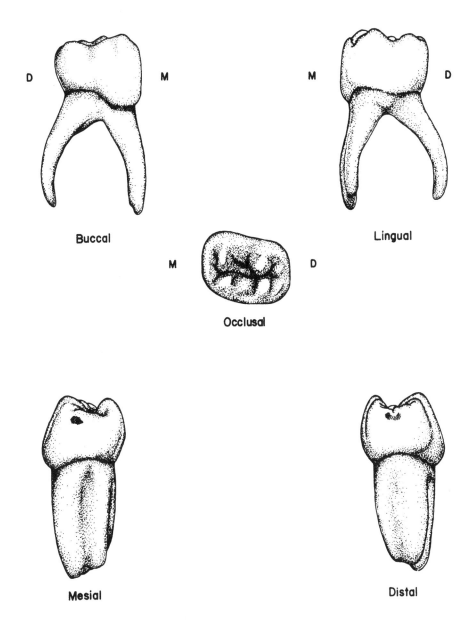

D   M

Buccal

M   D

Lingual

M   D

Occlusal

Mesial

Distal

MANDIBULAR RIGHT DECIDUOUS SECOND MOLAR

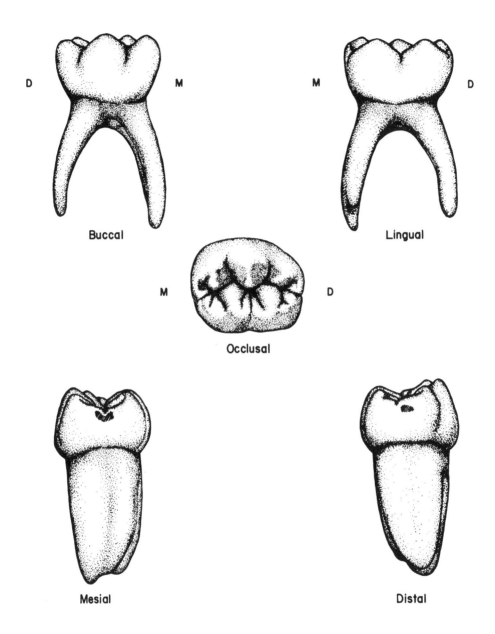

D   M

Buccal

M   D

Lingual

M   D

Occlusal

Mesial

Distal

UNIT # 11

I. **Reading Assignment:**

Unit # 11 (Development of the Teeth and Anomalies)

II. **Specific Objectives:**

At the completion of this unit, the student will be able to:

A.   Describe the four stages of morphologic tooth development prior to eruption, as well as the processes which occur during each stage, and the normal chronology of each stage, or select from a series of choices the correct information about the stages, when given a description or application.

B.   Describe the processes of eruption, resorption, exfoliation, and root completion, or select the correct response from a list regarding these processes or their normal chronology.

C.   Indicate a knowledge of the correct relationships of the permanent tooth buds to the roots of their deciduous predecessors by describing them, or choosing the correct information about them from a series of choices.

D.   Describe, or select from a list, the correct interpretation of the role played by the permanent first molars in the development of occlusion.

E.   Indicate the normal eruption sequence, or order, for deciduous and permanent teeth, by listing, or selecting from a list, the proper sequences.

F.   Describe the five stages of physiologic tooth development, as well as the processes which occur during each stage, and the normal chronology of each stage, or select from a series of choices the correct information about the stages, when given a description or application.

G.   Define any of the new terms, for example: enamel cuticle, Hertwig's sheath, ankylosis, active and passive eruption, etc., or select the proper definition, or application thereof, from a list, when given the term or a description or application.

H.   Identify from a given diagram or description of a dentition stage, the approximate age of the patient, or identify the number of teeth normally present at any given age.

I.   Indicate a knowledge of any of the anomalies, by defining or describing them, or by selecting the correct information about the anomaly or its features from a list, when given all, or significant portions of the etiology, clinical or x-ray manifestations, implications, or alternative names. Further, the student will be able to make comparisons between the various anomalies studied.

The student is also responsible for any material which was to have been mastered in previous units.

DEVELOPMENT OF THE TEETH AND ANOMALIES

I. **Development of the Teeth:**

A. Introduction:

1. The development of the dental structures is intimately related to the dentist's ability to properly predicate a thorough treatment plan for many patients. It is thus with total patient treatment that this overview of development is concerned.

2. Previously, when content has overlapped that of another course, present or future, the authors have elected to profile only the main points. So it is with this section on development; the salient features have been highlighted, with no effort made to reproduce the detail which the student should receive in histology, or related studies.

3. It should be pointed out that any development dates or patterns of eruption, when described as "normal" are only "average", or "most common". In reality, there is considerable variation in their range. As with other body growth patterns, if an individual is early or late in one phase of development, it is likely that other developmental phases will follow the same pattern.

B. Development of the Dental Organ:

As early as the second month of fetal life, the development of the deciduous teeth may first become evident. The transition from the earliest beginnings of the dental organ through its completion will be outlined in morphologic terms.

1. Dental lamina and Bud stage - At about six weeks of prenatal life, an epithelial thickening occurs in the region where the teeth will form. This thickening is termed the dental lamina. Shortly after the dental lamina differentiates, twenty tooth buds begin to appear on the dental lamina in the approximate location of the twenty primary teeth. The individual tooth buds are somewhat round, or ovoid, and this stage is appropriately known as the bud stage.

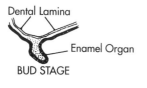

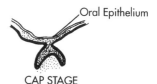

2. Cap stage - As further development takes place, the generally round form of the bud is altered. The basal portion invaginates, and the structure thus formed gives the appearance of a cap, and hence this phase is termed the cap stage.

3. Bell stage - As the concavity in the basal area of the cap continues to deepen, development of the tooth enters the bell stage. As this stage nears completion, the form of the tooth's crown can be recognized, and the dentinoenamel junction is identifiable. During this time, most of the crown's dentin and enamel is laid down. During the latter portion of the bell stage, the dental lamina connection with the deciduous tooth begins to break down, and eventually disintegrates. As this portion of the dental lamina disappears, the bud of the succedaneous tooth is forming from it.

Dental Lamina

BELL STAGE

4. Root development - When enamel and dentin deposition have formed the area of the cementoenamel junction, the bell stage is regarded as ending, and the root development stage begins. The enamel organ then proliferates a structure known as Hertwig's sheath, from which the root structure is formed. The dentin and cementum of the root are then deposited.

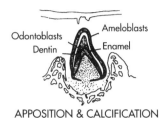

APPOSITION & CALCIFICATION

5. Chronology - The chronology of initiation of the tooth buds from the dental lamina occurs in three phases, over a total time period of about 5 1/2 years.

a. Deciduous dentition - As previously indicated, development of all deciduous teeth is initiated during the first few months of fetal life.

b. Succedaneous teeth - All the permanent successors to the deciduous teeth begin to form in a time range between five fetal months for the central incisors, to about 10 months after birth for the second premolars.

c. Non-succedaneous permanent teeth - The initiation of the permanent molars occurs in a time period between four fetal months for the first molars to approximately five years for the third molars.

C. Eruption:

1. Prior to the complete calcification of its root, the tooth normally originates eruption by pushing through the mucous membrane cover of the alveolar process, and into the oral cavity. The eruption process is considered complete when the tooth contacts its opponent(s) in the opposite jaw member. In reality, the term eruption involves two entities:

Enamel

Dentin

ERUPTION

a. Active eruption - Active eruption is the process just described, from the tooth's entry into the oral cavity, to its contact with an antagonist in the opposing arch.

b. Passive eruption - Passive eruption is the continuing process of adaptation of the tooth to changing incisal and occlusal relationships, after active eruption has ended. This adjustment to attritional wear and changing locations of adjacent and opposing teeth, continues throughout the life of the tooth. In fact, many times when a tooth has been lost, the antagonist(s) will supraerupt into the space, and beyond the normal occlusal plane.

2. When the tooth erupts, a keratinous, membrane-like enamel cuticle envelopes the anatomical crown. This structure, also known as Nasmyth's membrane, is soon abraded away over most of its extent.

3. Deciduous eruption pattern - The first deciduous teeth to emerge are the mandibular central incisors at about six months after birth. They are followed shortly thereafter by the mandibular lateral and maxillary central incisors. It is interesting to note that one in every several thousand infants enters the world with a tooth, or teeth, most often poorly developed mandibular incisors. At approximately two years of age, the average child erupts the deciduous maxillary

189

second molars, and thus has the function of all the deciduous teeth. This is an appropriate time to review the eruption pattern for the deciduous dentition which is presented in the first unit.

D.   Root completion:

As described previously, the root apex is funnel shaped shortly after eruption. Root formation is thus not complete until additional dentin deposition reduces the funnel shaped opening to a constricted foramen. At age 3, root formation has ended for all deciduous teeth. The time lag between eruption and root completion for the deciduous teeth is thus about one year, and the development tables reveal the time differential for permanent teeth.

ROOT COMPLETED

E.   Position of Developing Permanent Teeth:

All the while that the child is in the deciduous dentition stage, the permanent teeth are beginning, and continuing, their growth process. At this time, the development charts for permanent teeth should be reviewed to verify the beginnings of calcification and enamel completion dates. Remember that the time when the tooth bud first differentiates from the dental lamina is always prior to the initiation of calcification. Normally the succedaneous tooth buds exhibit a consistent relationship to the roots of the deciduous teeth they are to replace. The permanent incisor and canine buds are found in a position just lingual to the roots of their deciduous predecessors, while the premolar buds are located in the root furcation of the deciduous molars. The permanent molars are not succedaneous teeth, and their buds develop from the dental lamina in the alveolar process distal to the deciduous dentition.

F.   Late Deciduous Stage and Role of the Permanent First Molars:

1.   By approximately five years of age, growth of the mandible and maxilla has created more space for the permanent teeth which are soon to erupt. This extra space often results in the creation of <u>diastemas</u>, or spaces between adjacent teeth, usually in the anterior segment of the arches. Another suggested cause for the diastemas at this stage of development is the pressure exerted from the lingual by the developing permanent anterior teeth. The greater space in the arches also allows room for the entry of the first molars distal to the deciduous dentition.

2. The mandibular first molar is normally the first permanent tooth to emerge, at about age six, thus ending the deciduous dentition stage, and initiating the mixed dentition stage. The maxillary first molars follow shortly thereafter, and the four first molars are considered to be the cornerstones in the development of occlusion of the permanent dentition. Because they erupt first, and because of their strategic location in the arches, the relationship of the maxillary and mandibular first molars to each other has a significant influence on the occlusion of the permanent dentition. In addition, they serve as a guide for the eruption of the other permanent teeth, particularly the other molars. If any of the deciduous teeth are lost prematurely, the permanent first molar in that quadrant has a tendency to tilt or "drift" mesially, thus reducing the space available for the permanent canines and premolars. This condition changes the first molar's relationship with its antagonist(s), and may result in impaction of permanent teeth, or crowding and malocclusion of the permanent dental mechanism.

G. Resorption and Exfoliation:

  1. Resorption:

    a. Shortly after the permanent first molars appear, the permanent mandibular central incisors are scheduled to erupt. However, before this can occur, the deciduous predecessors must be shed, or exfoliated. The process by which the root of the deciduous tooth is "melted away" is termed resorption.

    b. Generally, resorption begins at the apex and moves toward the cervical line. Current thought ascribes the reason for the initiation and progression of resorption to be pressure from the permanent tooth crown against the deciduous root. The actual process is due to osteoclastic activity.

    c. The resorption phase normally begins at least a year prior to exfoliation. Thus, the period between the completion of the root for the second deciduous molars (about 3 years of age), and the initiation of resorption for some deciduous incisors (before age 5), is less than two years.

  2. Exfoliation - When the root structure of the deciduous tooth is almost entirely resorbed, the remaining crown becomes so loosened that it is lost. This phenomenon is known as exfoliation. Exfoliation usually occurs symmetrically, with the same teeth of the right and left sides being lost at about the same time. Mandibular teeth generally precede the same maxillary teeth in exfoliation, with the exception of the second molars, where all four are lost simultaneously. The same series of events occurs for all the deciduous teeth over a range of approximately six years, when the mixed dentition period ends with the exfoliation of the deciduous second molars at about age 12.

  3. Incomplete resorption - Occasionally, root resorption is only partial, and the deciduous tooth does not exfoliate. In this situation, the permanent tooth must erupt in an abnormal position, or be entirely blocked from entry. If this aberrant feature is present, it is the responsibility of the practitioner to diagnose it, and perform the customary treatment, which is extraction of the offending deciduous tooth.

  4. Ankylosis - Occasionally, the root structure of the deciduous tooth becomes "fused" to the surrounding alveolar bone. When this happens, any further eruption ceases, the tooth becomes "fixed" in position, and resorption cannot progress naturally. This condition is termed ankylosis, and occurs most often with the deciduous molars. The presence of an ankylosed tooth precludes the proper eruption of the succedaneous tooth, and so the ankylosed tooth must be surgically removed as soon as it is diagnosed.

H. Permanent Eruption Pattern:

The normal eruption pattern for the permanent teeth is found in Unit # 1, and will not be reproduced here. Furthermore, the normal dates of the various stages of permanent tooth development have been previously presented in the individual tooth units, and likewise will not be duplicated here. Please review these sequences and dates.

II. Anomalies:

A. Introduction:

  1. With the normal features of the teeth and their development as background, this final section is devoted to the etiology and description of some of the most common abnormalities of teeth, and tooth form. The term, anomaly, implies abnormality, as opposed to the normal range in variation of form. Even though

it may be only an academic question, it is sometimes difficult to differentiate between anomalies and extreme variations in morphology.

2. In many cases, it is difficult to intelligently discuss dental anomalies without pinpointing the stage of tooth development when the abnormality was manifest. In order to more accurately discuss the stages of development, a somewhat different classifying scheme, based on physiologic processes, as compared to morphologic stages, is briefly presented. These stages show a considerable overlap in time.

a. <u>Initiation</u> - The initiation process includes the dental lamina and bud stages, and affects the presence or absence of tooth buds.

b. <u>Proliferation</u> - Proliferation occurs during the bud, cap, and bell stages, and influences the general size and proportions of the tooth.

c. <u>Histodifferentiation</u> - This process takes place from the advanced cap stage through the bell stage, and essentially involves the formation of potential enamel and dentin forming cells.

d. <u>Morphodifferentiation</u> - The shape and size of the tooth is determined during this process, which takes place during the bud, cap, and bell stages. Thus, a disturbance during morphodifferentiation may influence the size and shape of a tooth, but have no effect on the enamel and dentin forming process.

e. <u>Apposition</u> - This process is active during the bell stage through the completion of the root, and involves the regular laying down of the enamel and dentin.

3. The general etiology of most dental anomalies can be ascribed to hereditary and congenital factors, or to developmental and metabolic disturbances. The stage of development, along with the length of the effect, are important factors influencing the final form of the anomaly, as well as which teeth are affected.

4. The permanent dentition is much more prone to abnormality than the deciduous teeth, and this may be partially explained by the position of the permanent tooth buds on the dental lamina, when compared to the primary tooth buds.

5. It is important to recognize that all anomalies are somewhat rare occurrences. Thus, it is often difficult to describe their frequencies, and they are usually compared in relative terms. None of the anomalies is present very often, but some are relatively more common than others.

B. Abnormal numbers of teeth:

1. Introduction:

The presence of an abnormal number of teeth, either more or less than usual, is almost always the result of some type of disturbance during the initiation process (dental lamina and bud stage) of tooth development. The disturbance is most often hereditary in nature.

2. <u>Anodontia</u> - Although this term literally signifies a "complete lack of teeth", its meaning has come to include any missing teeth, even if but one. Maybe a preferable term is <u>hypodontia</u>, which denotes agenesis of one or more teeth. Teeth which are impacted are not considered to be missing.

a. <u>Total anodontia</u> - This label implies a complete absence of teeth, but since that condition is extremely rare, with only a handful of reported cases, it has come to mean a large number of missing teeth. The etiology of total anodontia involves a sex-linked genetic trait which results in an ectodermal defect, and so structures such as hair, and sebaceous and sweat glands, are also abnormal. Except in the very rare cases mentioned, most or all of the primary teeth are present, while a lesser number of permanent teeth are found.

b. <u>Partial anodontia</u> - Generally speaking, partial anodontia involves but one, or a few, missing teeth, and is the result of hereditary factors which preclude the initiation of the tooth buds of affected teeth. It has been suggested that the dental lamina may fall below a certain threshold size for the forming of an individual tooth. The actual frequency has been shown to vary among population groups, but it can be generally stated that somewhere in the neighborhood of 5% of individuals exhibit one or more missing teeth. In order of greatest occurrence, the most commonly missing permanent teeth are the maxillary and mandibular third molars, the maxillary lateral incisor, and the mandibular second premolar. From an evolutionary standpoint, there is a trend toward less human teeth, and these most often missing teeth are considered by many to be vestigial in nature, while the least often missing teeth, the canines, are considered the most stable. Anodontia is quite rare in the deciduous dentition, but when present, almost always involves the mandibular central incisor.

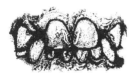

PARTIAL ANODONTIA
(MISSING MAXILLARY LATERAL INCISORS)

3. <u>Supernumerary (accesssory) teeth</u>:

a. The term, supernumerary, indicates an excessive number of teeth which are normal in morphological respects. However, since these "extra" teeth often do not resemble any normal tooth in size or shape, many authorities prefer to use the term "accessory" rather than supernumerary. The two terms will be used interchangeably here.

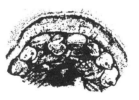

SUPERNUMERARY TOOTH
(PREMOLAR SHAPED)

b. Accessory teeth usually result when extra tooth buds differentiate from the dental lamina, and thus the etiology is considered to be genetic. Both deciduous and permanent dentitions may exhibit supernumerary teeth.

c. Accessory teeth have been found in various positions in the dental arches, but the vast majority of the permanent dentition specimens are found in either of two locations: between the maxillary central incisors (called <u>mesiodens</u>), or in the third molar regions (<u>distodens</u>). The only other area of significant involvement is, as might be expected, the mandibular second premolar area. However, many of the accessory teeth found in other areas resemble premolars. With the similar etiology, it is not surprising that the

193

areas commonly involved in supernumerary teeth are also the most frequent sites of partial anodontia. The frequency of supernumerary teeth is less than that of anodontia, and one study identified the condition in 1-2% of the general population.

C. Abnormal Size of Teeth:

1. Introduction:

Normally, an individual's teeth vary in size directly with their general face and body size. Therefore, large, or small teeth, when found in this context, are not considered to be abnormal. Furthermore, it is very rare for all of a person's teeth to be abnormal in size, since this anomaly is usually limited to a single tooth, or a few teeth of the same type. This condition is thought to be the result of a disturbance during morphodifferentiation in the bell stage, with a genetic etiology.

2. Macrodontia (Gigantism):

a. True macrodontia - In the rare case of pituitary gigantism, all the teeth are abnormally large.

b. False macrodontia - More commonly, individual teeth are excessive in size, and those most frequently involved are incisors, canines, and mandibular third molars.

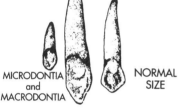

MICRODONTIA and MACRODONTIA   NORMAL SIZE

3. Microdontia (Dwarfism)

a. True microdontia - Pituitary dwarfs may exhibit true microdontia, when all the teeth are abnormally small.

b. False microdontia - It is much more common to find microdontia in individual teeth, and those most frequently involved are the maxillary lateral incisors (peg lateral), and the maxillary third molars.

D. Abnormal Shape of Teeth:

1. Introduction:

The presence of abnormal crown and root shapes and contours is most often the result of disturbances during the morphodifferentiation and appositional stages of tooth development.

2. Taurodontism - This condition of premolars and molars of both dentitions is characterized by a crown which occupies a much greater proportion of the total tooth bulk than is normal. The CEJ shows no constriction, the furcation is found in the apical half of the tooth, and the floor of the pulp chamber is likewise displaced apically. Since the size of the tooth itself is normal, the increased extent of the crown and pulp chamber occur at the expense of the root and pulp canals. The condition may be unilateral or bilateral. Taurodontism is usually diagnosed by x-ray, and is clinically significant only if root canal therapy is necessary. The etiology is hereditary, often in conjunction with other syndromes.

3. Dilaceration - This abnormality reveals a distortion of the root and crown from their normally linear relationship. The cause is most often a traumatic injury, or pressure, to the area of a developing tooth, resulting in a displacement of the already formed portion of the tooth.

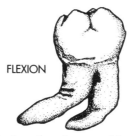

DILACERATION

4. Flexion - As contrasted to dilaceration, flexion involves a distortion of the root portion only. The etiology is normally the same for both, but occurs later in the development cycle in flexion. Many teeth exhibit curvatures and deflections of their roots, but they are not considered abnormal unless the bends are sharp.

FLEXION

5. Gemination - Gemination is thought to be caused by the incomplete splitting of a single tooth germ. The result is a tooth which is wide mesiodistally, and which has an incisal notch if it is an anterior tooth. It normally has a single root with a common pulp cavity. The two components of the gemination may be nearly equal in size, or one portion may be rudimentary in both size and shape, when compared to the other portion. The geminated tooth is most often an incisor. The term twinning is used to identify a situation where gemination has been complete, resulting in two identical teeth, and thus an additional tooth in the dentition.

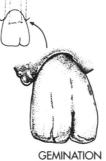

GEMINATION

6. Fusion - This anomaly is considered to be the result of a union of two adjacent tooth buds. The exact etiology is not known, but is thought to be either heredi- tary or from pressure exerted when two tooth buds are in very close proximity. The two portions are always united through the enamel and dentin, and occa- sionally even the pulp. The fusion usually concerns only the crowns, but on occasion involves both crown and root, in which case the cementum of the two portions is also united. Fusion is also usually found in anterior teeth. Unlike

gemination, there are normally two identifiable pulp cavities. It is further differentiated from gemination by an apparently greater degree of separation of the two portions. And, unlike gemination there is one less dental unit than normal in the dentition, if the fused tooth is counted as one unit. Fusion is more often found in the deciduous teeth, and may be unilateral or bilateral. Because they are sometimes difficult to differentiate clinically, the term "double tooth" has been suggested to include all geminations, twinnings, and fusions.

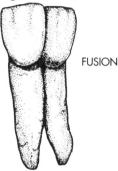

FUSION

7.   Concrescence - This entity involves the union of the root structure of two or more teeth through cementum only. The teeth involved are originally separated, but join because of excessive cementum deposition of one or both teeth. This condition is most common in the permanent molars, particularly those of the maxillary arch, and logically occurs when the roots are in close proximity. It differs from fusion, because it is not a union between two tooth germs during development, but normally occurs following eruption, and it never involves enamel and dentin. It should be obvious that concrescence would be a hazard to any extraction procedure of the teeth involved.

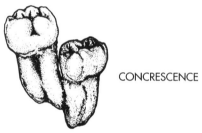

CONCRESCENCE

8.   Segmented root - This anomaly is caused by some disturbance during root development, and results in two separated root segments. The specific etiology is thought to be a break in Hertwig's sheath, temporarily halting dentinogenesis, so that if the formative process continues, the two root portions are separated.

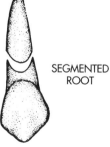

SEGMENTED
ROOT

9. Dwarfed roots - This condition exists when normal sized crowns have abnormally short roots. The crowns of these teeth are also abnormal in contour, exhibiting a greater incisocervical convexity of the labial surface. Normally, dwarfed roots are found only in the anterior teeth, most commonly the maxillary central incisors. The condition is quite often bilateral. It is also thought to have a hereditary etiology. These teeth may be lost at an early age simply because of passive eruption, or periodontal disease. This anomaly should not be confused with the shortened roots and blunted apices of teeth, occasionally observed radiographically following orthodontic treatment, and caused by excessive pressures during tooth movement.

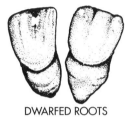

DWARFED ROOTS

10. Hypercementosis - As its name suggests, this condition results in excessive cementum formation around the root of a tooth, and is most often associated with the roots of permanent molars. It normally is not associated with any stage of tooth development, but rather occurs after eruption. The etiology may involve one of several sources, including trauma, local or systemic metabolic disturbance, or most commonly, chronic inflammation of the pulp.

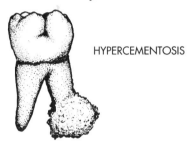

HYPERCEMENTOSIS

11. Accessory cusps and roots - This group constitutes the most commonly observed dental anomalies, and may be attributed to hereditary or developmental causes during the morphodifferentiation process.

a. Accessory cusps - Extra cusps, or tubercles, are most often found in molars, and third molars in particular. They also occur as an incisal extension of the cingulum in maxillary anteriors. In the maxillary incisors, this occurrence is known as talon cusp. The crown of the affected incisor may give the appearance of a Phillips screwdriver. The etiology of talon cusp is not known, but is probably hereditary, since it often occurs in conjunction with other anomalies.

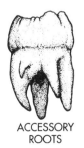

ACCESSORY ROOTS

b. Accessory roots - Most often, extra roots are found on teeth which undergo root development after birth, and so the etiology is considered to be trauma, pressure, or metabolic disease. The third molars most often exhibit accessory roots, but they may be found on any tooth in the mouth, although rarely in the maxillary anterior teeth. Maxillary first premolars with three roots and mandibular anterior teeth with two roots are also found. As might be expected, their presence is quite often a hazard in extraction procedures.

197

12. <u>Missing cusps</u> - Cusps of permanent posterior teeth are occasionally absent. Those most often missing are the most diminutive, good examples of which are the lingual cusp of the mandibular first premolar, the distolingual cusp of maxillary molars, and the distal cusp of mandibular first molars.

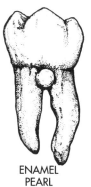

13. <u>Enamel pearls</u> - Also known as enamelomas, or enamel drops, they are found attached to the root surfaces of teeth, in the form of small, spherical nodules of enamel surrounding a dentin core. Their specific site is usually in the furcation area of molars. Because of the root anatomy, this means their location is most likely to be the buccal and lingual of mandibular molars, and the mesial and distal of maxillary molars. They are thought to be the result of aberrant enamel deposition on the root initiated by Hertwig's sheath. The enameloma appears as a round radiopaque mass on x-rays. They may be of clinical significance in the predisposition to, or severity of, periodontal disease. This abnormality has about a 2% incidence in the general population.

ENAMEL
PEARL

14. <u>Hutchinson's teeth</u> - This anomaly is often classified with hypoplastic defects, because it is a type of enamel dysplasia, but we will consider it in this section of abnormal form. The condition is due to prenatal syphilis. Specifically, its etiology involves the disturbance of calcification by the treponema organism during ameloblastic morphodifferentiation. Since the incisors and first molars are the only permanent teeth at this stage of development, they exhibit the effects. Primary teeth are not normally involved. The incisor crowns exhibit a screwdriver shape, usually with a deep notch on the incisal edge. The first molars have a mulberry appearance, with gnarled enamel, and poorly developed cusps. The dental significance is primarily esthetic.

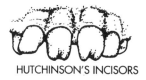

HUTCHINSON'S INCISORS

15. <u>Dens in dente</u> - This condition occurs when the enamel organ becomes invaginated in a specific area on the crown of the tooth, and the normally external structures of enamel and dentin become reversed inside the pulp cavity. This creates an x-ray appearance of a small tooth within a tooth, hence the name dens in dente. It is rare in the posterior teeth, and is most commonly found in the permanent maxillary lateral incisor. In these teeth, the invagination leaves a defect in the lingual surface, in the form of an opening, or lingual pit, which leads to an enamel and dentin enclosed pulp cavity. As a result, it easily becomes carious and eventually may cause pain. Normally, the condition is evident in radiographs.

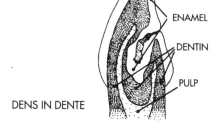

ENAMEL

DENTIN

PULP

DENS IN DENTE

16. Odontoma:

    a. Introduction - An odontoma is really not an anomaly of shape, but rather a benign tumor. It is included in this section for lack of a better location. The odontoma is a growth of calcified dental tissues, involving structures of both ectodermal (enamel) and mesodermal (dentin, cementum, and pulp) origin. There are two basic types, both of which evidently result from developmental disturbances of the dental lamina, or follicle, by trauma or infection.

    b. Complex odontoma - This growth consists of one mass of calcified dental tissues, and may be attached to a normal tooth, or located separately in the alveolar bone. It does not exhibit any definite dental form.

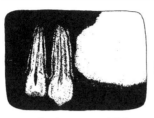

COMPLEX
ODONTOMA
(RADIOGRAPHIC VIEW)

    c. Compound odontoma - This type of odontoma also consists of the calcified tissues of a tooth, but in contrast to the complex type, these tissues are arranged in the shape of a recognizable tooth form. There may be one or more of these tooth forms, sometimes with almost perfect similarity to a normal tooth, and sometimes resembling more rudimentary dental forms.

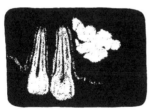

COMPOUND ODONTOMA
(RADIOGRAPHIC VIEW)

E. Abnormal Calcification and Apposition:

    1. Introduction:

This group of anomalies is the result of disturbances which affect enamel and dentin formation during the histodifferentiation and appositional processes. The resultant condition is dependent on the severity of the disturbance, the stage of matrix or calcification affected, as well as the length of the disturbance.

    2. Enamel dysplasia:

    a. Introduction - Enamel dysplasia is a catchall label, and encompasses all enamel development abnormalities. The etiologic agents may be local, systemic, or hereditary in nature. Clinically, enamel dysplasias are characterized by bands, ridges, or pitted areas of discolored enamel. The size of the affected areas is directly related to the length and severity of the etiologic disturbance. Only teeth undergoing enamel formation at the time of disturbance are affected. The two general types of enamel dysplasia include:

    i. Enamel hypoplasia - This type of enamel dysplasia occurs when the disturbance in development occurs during enamel matrix formation.

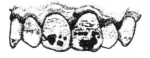

ENAMEL
HYPOPLASIA

ii. Enamel hypocalcification - The time of disturbance in hypo-calcification is later than for hypoplasia, and occurs during enamel matrix maturation.

b. Amelogenesis imperfecta - This type of enamel dysplasia has an hereditary cause. The defect may range from an almost complete absence of enamel, to enamel that was deposited, but failed to fully mature, depending on the stage at which the disturbance occurred. The crowns of teeth with this abnormality are subject to rampant caries, as well as excessive attrition. For this reason, these teeth are rarely seen as late as adult life. They are also an esthetic consideration, since the crowns exhibit a surface roughness. The incidence of this dysplasia has been reported as about one in 14,000.

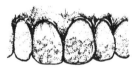

AMELOGENESIS
IMPERFECTA

c. Dental fluorosis (Mottled enamel) - The intake of excessively high levels of fluoride ion during the enamel calcification period is responsible for this type of enamel dysplasia. It is considered to be a hypocalcification problem, since sufficient enamel matrix is normally present. The clinical appearance originally reveals chalky white bands or areas, which usually become pigmented in a brown or yellow fashion. Because of the etiology, these teeth are usually quite resistant to caries, which is in contrast to the other forms of enamel dysplasia. However, they may be a severe esthetic detriment to the patient.

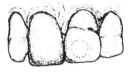

DENTAL FLUOROSIS

d. Focal hypomaturation - This entity is similar in etiology to the other enamel dysplasias. Clinically, it appears as a chalky white and opaque area which is clearly defined, usually in a circular shape on the facial surface. The enamel is particularly susceptible to caries. If, as is normally true, it is found in the anterior teeth, it is an esthetic consideration also.

FOCAL
HYPOMATURATION

e. Turner's teeth - This condition is found in individual teeth, as a result of local etiologic factors. The most common of these specific causes involves injury to the developing permanent tooth follicle through extraction procedures of the deciduous tooth, or disturbance from periapical infection of a diseased deciduous tooth pulp. Because of the different etiology, these clinically unesthetic areas are not generally symmetrical like most of the other anomalies of this group.

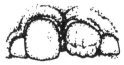

TURNER'S
TEETH

3. Dentinal dysplasia:

a. Introduction - The dentin dysplasias disturb dentin matrix formation and calcification during histodifferentiation and appositional processes. They are similar in all aspects to enamel dysplasias, except that the dental tissue involved is dentin rather than enamel.

b. Tetracycline staining - It has been documented that the administration of the wide-spectrum antibiotic tetracyclines, either to the mother during certain prenatal periods, or to the infant, may impart an intrinsic color change to the dentin of teeth undergoing mineralization. Both primary and permanent teeth may be affected, and the extent and location of any individual teeth is related to the time and duration of the antibiotic therapy. The affected teeth may originally exhibit a yellowish cast but with time change to a grayish or even purplish color.

c. Dentinogenesis imperfecta - This abnormality results from the genetic disturbance of dentin formation, and is the dentinal counterpart of amelogenesis imperfecta. The crown of the tooth exhibits an unesthetic clinical appearance of opalescence, which is bluish-brown in color, and thus the condition is also known as opalescent dentin. The pulp chamber of these teeth may be entirely obliterated during development. The enamel is normal, but fractures easily, because of the lack of sound underlying dentinal support. Therefore, these teeth are weaker, and subject to greater attrition than normal teeth.

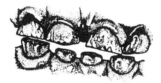

HEREDITARY
DENTINOGENESIS
IMPERFECTA

F. Treatment:

Since your dental background is admittedly limited, a discussion of the normal treatment of the various anomalies has been omitted. Some of the abnormalities require no treatment at all, but many of them require very challenging, imaginative, and highly skilled treatment. However, before any treatment should be attempted, an accurate diagnosis of the abnormality, and its implications, is imperative.

INDEX

A

Accessory teeth *(see* Supernumerary teeth)
Adodontia, 192-93
  partial, 193
  total, 192-93
Age: and pulp cavity changes, 139
Agenesis, 49
Alveolar process, 12
Alveolus, 12
Amelogenesis imperfecta, 200
Anastomosis
  definition, 138
  illustration, 148
Anatomic considerations: of form and
  function, 23-38
Anatomy
  dental
    comparative, 23-24
    general, 11-12
  occlusal, 37
  oral, general, 11-12
  pulp cavity, 137-38
Ankylosis, 191
Anomalies, 191-201
  canine
    mandibular, 65
    maxillary, 63
  incisor, central
    mandibular, 52
    maxillary, 46
  incisor, lateral
    mandibular, 53
    maxillary, 49
  molar, first
    mandibular, 126
    maxillary, 107
  molar, second
    mandibular, 130
    maxillary, 110
  molar, third
    mandibular, 131
    maxillary, 111
  numbers of teeth, 192-94
  premolar, first
    mandibular, 91
    maxillary, 78
  premolar, second
    mandibular, 96
    maxillary, 81

  shape of teeth, 194-99
  size of teeth, 194
  treatment, 201
Anterior teeth, 12
  crown surface form, 29
  heights of contour on facial and lingual
    surfaces, 34
  line angles, 14
  lobes, 25-26
  point angles of, 15
  surfaces, 13
Antrum, 78, 81
Apical foramen
  definition, 138
  illustrations, 148-49
Apical thirds, 17
Apposition, 192
  abnormal, 199-201
Arch(es), 2
Arch position, permanent teeth
  canine, 59
    mandibular, 63
    maxillary, 59
  incisor, central
    mandibular, 49
    maxillary, 42
  incisor, lateral
    mandibular, 52
    maxillary, 46
  molar, first
    mandibular, 118
    maxillary, 101
  molar, second
    mandibular, 126
    maxillary, 108
  molar, third
    mandibular, 130
    maxillary, 110
  premolar, first
    mandibular, 86
    maxillary, 71
  premolar, second
    mandibular, 91
    maxillary, 78
Axial position, 28

203

F

Facial height: of contour, 33-34
Facial surface, 13
Faciolingual section: of pulp cavity,139, 150
Federal Dentaire Internationale numbering
    system, 10
Fissure: linguogingival, 48
Flexion, 195
Fluorosis: dental, 200
Focal hypomaturation, 200
Foramen *(see* Apical foramen)
Form
    anatomic considerations of, 23-39
    canine, 59
    physiologic considerations of, 23-39
    premolar, 70
Fossa
    central *(see* Central fossa)
    definition, 20
    distal *(see* Distal fossa)
    distolingual *(see* Distolingual fossa)
    lingual, permanent incisors, 41
        maxillary central, 44
    mesial *(see* Mesial fossa)
    mesiolingual *(see* Mesiolingual fossa)
    molar, first
        mandibular, deciduous, 175
        mandibular, permanent, 124
        maxillary, deciduous, 173
        maxillary, permanent, 105-106
    molar, second, permanent mandibular,
    129
    premolar, first
        mandibular, 90
        maxillary, 76
    premolar, second, mandibular, 94, 95
    triangular *(see* Triangular fossa)
Function
    anatomic considerations of, 23-39
    physiologic considerations of, 23-39
Furcation, 77
Fusion, 195-96

G

Gemination, 195
Gigantism *(see* Macrodontia)
Gingiva: definition, 12
Gingival
    crest, 35
    embrasures, 31-32
    line, 35
    margin, 35
    tissue, 31

Grooves
Buccal *(see* Buccal groove)
    central *(see* Central, groove)
    cusp of Carabelli, 103
    developmental *(see* Developmental groove)
    distobuccal, mandibular first molar, 119-20
    distolingual, 100, 106
    disto-occlusal, 173
    lingual *(see* Lingual groove)
    linguogingival *(see* Linguogingival groove)
    longitudinal *(see* Longitudinal groove)
    marginal *(see* Marginal groove)
    molar, first
        mandibular, deciduous, 175-76
        mandibular, permanent, 124
        maxillary, deciduous, 173
        maxillary, permanent, 106-07
    molar, second, permanent mandibular,
        129
    premolar, first
        mandibular, 96
        maxillary, 76
    premolar, second, mandibular, 94, 95
    supplemental *(see* Supplemental groove)
    triangular *(see* Triangular groove)

H

Heart-shaped molar, 109-110, 114
Heights: of contour, facial and lingual, 33-34
Dentinogenesis imperfecta, 201
Hertwig's sheath, 189
Heterodont, 3
Histodifferentiation, 192
Homodont, 3
Hutchinson's incisors, 46, 198
Hypercementosis, 197
Hypocalcification: enamel, 200
Hypodontia, 192
Hypornaturation: focal, 200
Hypoplasia: enamel, 199

I

Imbrication lines, 43, 47, 61, 64, 72, 87
Impacted
    canine, maxillary, 63
    molar, third
        mandibular, 131
        maxillary, 111
Incisal
    edge, 13, 45, 48
    embrasures, 31-32
    ridge, 13, 45
    slopes, canine, comparison of newly
        erupted and worn, 68

first, maxillary, 73, 76
second, mandibular, 94
Mesial marginal ridge
incisor, maxillary central, 44
molar, first
mandibular, 121
maxillary, 124
premolar, first
mandibular, 90
maxillary, 95
Mesial pit
molar, first
mandibular, deciduous, 175
mandibular, permanent, 125
maxillary, deciduous, 173
maxillary, permanent, 106
molar, second, permanent mandibular,
129
premolar, first
mandibular, 90
maxillary, 76
premolar, second, mandibular, 94, 95
Mesial root, mandibular first molar
deciduous, 157
permanent, 125
Mesial surface
anterior teeth, 13
posterior teeth, 13
Mesial triangular fossa
molar, first
mandibular, deciduous, 175
mandibular, permanent, 124
maxillary, deciduous, 173
maxillary, permanent, 106
premolar
first, maxillary, 76
second, mandibular, 94
Mesiobuccal cusp, mandibular molar
first, 122-23
second, 128
Mesiobuccal developmental depression, first
premolar
mandibular, 87
maxillary, 72
Mesiobuccal groove: mandibular first molar,
119, 124
Mesiobuccal lobe
molar
mandibular, first, 26
mandibular second, 27
maxillary, 26
premolar, 25
Mesiobuccal root, 107

Mesiobuccal triangular groove
molar, first
mandibular, 125
maxillary, 106
molar, second, mandibular, 129
premolar, first
mandibular, 90
maxillary, 76
Mesiodens, 193
Mesiodistal section: of pulp cavity, 139, 150
Mesioincisal slope, 60, 64
Mesiolabial developmental depression, 25
canine, maxillary, 61
incisor, maxillary central, 43
Mesiolabial lobe, 25
Mesiolingual cusp
molar, first
mandibular, 123
maxillary, 105
molar, second, mandibular, 128
premolar, mandibular second, 92, 94
Mesiolingual developmental groove, 88, 90
Mesiolingual fossa, canine
mandibular, 64
maxillary, 61
Mesiolingual lobe
molar
mandibular, first, 26
maxillary, 26
premolar, 25
Mesiolingual triangular groove
molar, first
mandibular, 125
maxillary, 106
molar, second, mandibular, 129
premolar
first, maxillary, 76
second, mandibular, 94
Mesio-occlusal slope, first premolar
mandibular, 87
maxillary, 72
Microdontia, 194
false, 194
true, 194
Middle buccal lobe, 25
Middle labial lobe, 25
Middle thirds, 16-17
Midline, 2
Mid-sagittal plane, 2
Missing teeth (*see* Congenitally missing)
Molar
deciduous, 4
(*See also below*)

213

crown form, 28-29
posterior teeth, 13
proximal, 13
root, 13

T

Talon cusp, 46, 197
Taurodontism, 194
Teeth
  (*See also* Dentition)
  accessory *(see* Supernumerary teeth)
  anterior *(see* Anterior teeth)
  classification of, 4
  congenitally missing *(see* Congenitally
    missing)
  development of, 188-89
  "double tooth," 196
  Hutchinson's, 46, 198
  numbers of, abnormal, 192-93
  posterior *(see* Posterior teeth)
  shape, abnormal, 194-99
  size, abnormal, 194
  succedaneous, 5
  supernumerary *(see* Supernumerary teeth)
  surfaces, 13
  tritubercular, 24
  Turner's, 200
  wisdom *(see* Molar, third)
Tetracycline staining, 201
Thirds: of crown and root, 16-17
Tissue
  gingival, 31
  pulp *(see* Pulp, tissue)
Tooth *(see* Teeth)
Transverse ridge, 18, 20
  definition, 18
  molar, first
    mandibular, deciduous, 175
    mandibular, permanent, 124
    maxillary, deciduous, 173
    maxillary, permanent, 105
  molar, second, permanent mandibular,
    129
  premolar, first
    mandibular, 90
    maxillary, 75
  premolar, second, mandibular, 95
Trapezoidal shaped crowns, 28, 29
Triangular fossa
  distal *(see* Distal triangular fossa)
  mesial *(see* Mesial triangular fossa)
Triangular groove
  distobuccal *(see* Distobuccal triangular

    groove)
  distolingual *(see* Distolingual triangular
    groove)
  mesiobuccal *(see* Mesiobuccal triangular
    groove)
  mesiolingual *(see* Mesiolingual triangular
    groove)
Triangular ridge, 18, 20
  definition, 18
Triangular shaped crowns, 28, 29
Tritubercular tooth, 24
Tubercles: definition, 15
Turner's teeth, 200
Twinning, 195

U

Universal number
  deciduous teeth, 7-8
  permanent teeth *(see below)*
  system, 7-9
Universal number, permanent teeth, 7, 9
  canine
    mandibular, 63
    maxillary, 59
  incisor, central
    mandibular, 49
    maxillary, 42
  incisor, lateral
    mandibular, 52
    maxillary, 46
  molar, first
    mandibular, 118
    maxillary, 101
  molar, second
    mandibular, 126
    maxillary, 108
  molar, third
    mandibular, 130
    maxillary, 110
  premolar, first
    mandibular, 86
    maxillary, 71
  premolar, second
    mandibular, 91
    maxillary, 79

W

Wisdom teeth *(see* Molar, third)

PRONUNCIATION GUIDE

Anastomosis - (A nas ta mō' sis)

Agenesis - (Ā jen' a sis)

Alveolus - (Al vē' ō lus)

Ameloblast - (A mē' lō blast)

Amelogenesis - (A mē' lō jen' a sis)

Ankylosis - (An ka lō' sis)

Anodontia - (An ō don' sha)

Apical - (Āp' i kl)

Axial - (Ak' sē al)

Bifurcation - (Bī fur kā' shen)

Buccal - (Buck' l)

Carabelli - (Kair a bel' ē)

Cementum - (Si men' tum)

Cervical - (Sur' vi kl)

Cingulum - (Sin' gū lum)

Concrescence - (Kon kres' ns)

Congenital - (Kon jen' i tl)

Deciduous - (Di sij' oo wus)

Dens in Dente - (Denz) (in) (dent' ā)

Dentin - (Den' tin)

Dentinogenesis - (Den' tin ō jen' a sis)

Diastema - (Dī' a sta ma)

Dilaceration - (Dī' las ur ā shen)

Diphyodont - (Dī fī ō dont)

Distal - (Dis' tl)

Dysplasia - (Dis plā' zhē-a)

Embrasure - (Im brā' zher)

Enamel - (I nam' l)

Enameloma - (I nam' l ō ma)

Endodontia - (En dō don' sha)

Exfoliate - (Eks fō' lē āt)

Facial - (Fā' shl)

Flexion - (Flek' shen)

Fluorosis - (Floo' er ō sis)

Foramen - (For ā' men)

Fossa - (Faus' a)

Fusion - (Fū' zhen)

Gemination - (Jem' i nā shen)

Gingival - (Jin' ji vl)

Heterodont - (Het' ur ō dont)

Homodont - (Hō' mō dont)

Hypercementosis - (Hī' pur si' men tō sis)

Hypomaturation - (Hī' pō ma' chur ā shen)

Hypoplasia - (Hī' pō plā' zhē-a)

Imbrication - (Im bra kā' shen)

Impaction - (Im pak' shen)

Incisal - (In sī' zl)

Labial - (Lā' be l)

Lamination - (Lam' in ā shen)

Lingual - (Lin' gwel)

Longitudinal - (Lon ja too' di nl)

Macrodontia - (ma' krō don sha)

Mamelon - (Mam' a lon)

Mandibular - (Man dib' yoo lar)

Mastication - (Mas' ti kā shen)

Maxillary - (Mak' se ler ē)

Mesial - (Mē' zē el)

Microdontia - (Mī' krō don sha)

Monophyodont - (mo' nō fī ō dont)

Nasmyth - (Naz' mith)

Occlusal - (A kloo' zl)

Occlusion - (A kloo' zhen)

Odontoblast - (Ō don' tō blast)

Odontoma - (Ō don tō' ma)

Opalescent - (Ō pa les' nt)

Orifice - (Or' a fis)

Palatal - (Pal' a tl)

Periodontium - (Per ē ō don' she-um)

Polyphyodont - (Pol ē fī' ō dont)

Proximal - (Prok' se ml)

Resorption - (Rē sorp' shen)

Succedaneous - (Suk si dān' ē us)

Sulcus - (Sul kes)

Supernumerary - (Soo per noo' me rer ē)

Tubercle - (Too' bur kl)

Tritubercular - (Trī' too burk' yoo lar)